T0227758

Age–Period–Cohort Models

Models

Approaches and Analyses
with Aggregate Data

Chapman & Hall/CRC
Statistics in the Social and Behavioral Sciences Series

Aims and scope

Large and complex datasets are becoming prevalent in the social and behavioral sciences and statistical methods are crucial for the analysis and interpretation of such data. This series aims to capture new developments in statistical methodology with particular relevance to applications in the social and behavioral sciences. It seeks to promote appropriate use of statistical, econometric and psychometric methods in these applied sciences by publishing a broad range of reference works, textbooks and handbooks.

The scope of the series is wide, including applications of statistical methodology in sociology, psychology, economics, education, marketing research, political science, criminology, public policy, demography, survey methodology and official statistics. The titles included in the series are designed to appeal to applied statisticians, as well as students, researchers and practitioners from the above disciplines. The inclusion of real examples and case studies is therefore essential.

Chapman & Hall/CRC
Statistics in the Social and Behavioral Sciences Series

Age–Period–Cohort Models

Approaches and Analyses with Aggregate Data

Robert M. O'Brien

University of Oregon
Eugene, USA

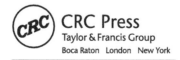

CRC Press
Taylor & Francis Group
Boca Raton London New York

CRC Press is an imprint of the
Taylor & Francis Group, an **informa** business

A CHAPMAN & HALL BOOK

CRC Press
Taylor & Francis Group
6000 Broken Sound Parkway NW, Suite 300
Boca Raton, FL 33487-2742

© 2015 by Taylor & Francis Group, LLC
CRC Press is an imprint of Taylor & Francis Group, an Informa business

No claim to original U.S. Government works

International Standard Book Number-13: 978-1-4665-5153-4 (Hardback)

Visit the Taylor & Francis Web site at
http://www.taylorandfrancis.com

and the CRC Press Web site at
http://www.crcpress.com

Contents

Preface

The separation of age effects from period effects from cohort effects is a key problem for any analysis involving one or more of these effects. Yet this problem is too often ignored. In a cross-sectional survey, the researcher may find that age is related to smoking behavior. This research controls for the effect of periods by examining only one period: limiting the period variance to zero and its "effect" to zero. The "obvious" cross-sectional "age effect" that results, however, could be a cohort effect or due to age and cohort effects, because in this cross-sectional design each age group represents a different birth cohort. An analogous problem occurs when examining a single age group across a number of periods or a single cohort across a number of ages. These situations involve omitted variables.

Often researchers design their studies with two of these three factors in mind. The researcher might begin with an age-by-period design, focus on how the age distribution has fluctuated in different periods, and come up with explanations for why different periods have affected the age distribution of tuberculosis, or favorability to same sex marriages, or suicides. Researchers using this design may well ignore the possible effects of cohorts. But those effects should not be ignored, since there is a confounding of the effects of age, period, and cohort: if we know the age and we know the period, we know the birth cohort. There is a linear dependency between the independent variables (Period – Age = Cohort).

In the aforementioned scenarios, researchers may not recognize that they face the age–period–cohort (APC) identification problem, but they most certainly do. Researchers who analyze the data explicitly taking into account age, period, and cohort effects are almost all cognizant of the identification problem in such models. They recognize that models including age, period, and cohort effects have a linear dependency.

This book is an introduction to the problem and strategies for modeling age, period, and cohort effects for aggregate-level data. These strategies range from constrained estimation to the use of age and/or period and/or cohort characteristics; from these factor-characteristic approaches to estimable functions; from estimable functions to variance decomposition. After a general and wide-ranging introductory chapter, Chapters 2 and 3 explicate the identification problem from an algebraic and a geometric perspective. They also discuss constrained regression. Chapters 4 through 6 provide some important strategies that give us information that does not directly depend on the constraints used in Chapters 2 and 3 to identify the APC model. Chapter 7 presents a specific empirical example in which I show how a combination of the approaches presented in this book can make a compelling case for particular age, period, and cohort effects.

The literature on APC models is extensive. In this book, I provide an introduction to part of this literature from the classic perspective by examining
APC models that use aggregate-level data. These data are of the type available in Vital Statistics, Uniform Crime Reports, or other government archives
that report the number of cases of homicides or marriages or mortality due
to tuberculosis by age group for different years. The same sort of analysis is
often conducted using repeated cross-sectional surveys that can be aggregated into age distributions and that were conducted during different time
periods. I focus on the problems and strategies used at this aggregate level
even though some approaches to APC models use data from both the individual level and aggregate level to estimate age, period, and cohort effects. In
Chapter 5 on variance decomposition approaches, I comment on such mixed-
level models. The design or plan of this book is presented at the end of the
introductory chapter (Chapter 1).

There are some key people to thank. William (Bill) Mason gave a talk at
the University of Oregon in the late 1980s on political alienation and relative
cohort size. It was the beginning of my interest in the APC perspective. His
presentation was so clear that even I could run the analysis he outlined in
his talk. Jean Stockard reignited my interest in APC analysis with a potential
explanation of a graph showing the epidemic of youth homicide that I had
shown her. We had the most fruitful publication collaboration in which I
have ever participated. Chris Winship, as editor of *Sociological Methods and
Research*, kept probing me with questions and asking for better explanations
of claims I was making in an article that was under review. He also insisted
that I and colleagues who would eventually comment on my article reach
the highest degree of civility—arguing to the point and not the person. As
a coeditor of a sociological journal myself (*Sociological Perspectives*), I can
only work toward such qualities. Then there are the many talented instructors
who "brought me along" when I was an undergraduate at Pomona College.
When I entered college, I was more focused on basketball than academics.
The professors at the University of Wisconsin invested their time in me as
well, where the focus was on making me a professional sociologist and, yes,
on the value of good old Midwestern empiricism. Two people suggested that
I write a book before I thought of it: my eldest son Josh O'Brien, and Chris
Winship. Then, I was contacted by Chapman & Hall and the rest is history,
well personal history.

Author

Robert M. O'Brien is a professor emeritus of sociology at the University of Oregon. He specializes in criminology and quantitative methods. He has published extensively in both areas. In semiretirement, he coedits *Sociological Perspectives* with James R. Elliott and works on research projects such as this book.

1

Introduction to the Age, Period, and Cohort Mix

A knowledge of epidemiological history, combined with a firm grasp of the statistical method were as essential parts of the outfit of the investigator in that field as was a grounding in bacteriology.

Major Greenwood (Hardy and Magnello 2004:214)

1.1 Introduction

In the context of this book, the opening quote calls for a grounding in a substantive area such as epidemiology, demography, or one of the social sciences and statistical methods appropriate to the problem. More explicitly, in this context it calls for substantive knowledge about the potential effects of age, period, and cohort on a substantive variable within a field and the appropriate statistical methods for dealing with age, period, and cohort relationships. I will not provide a substantive grounding in any one of these fields or even provide a comprehensive review of the literature on age, period, and cohort models within one of these fields. My objective is different.

This book focuses on obtaining a deep understanding of the statistical opportunities and complications associated with age, period, and cohort analysis, and using that understanding to evaluate how several of the most common methods in the literature are related to one another and how they can be utilized to obtain answers to some of the questions concerning the relationships of age, period, and cohort to substantively important variables. This deep understanding should help readers to evaluate new methods that they discover in the literature and to use those methods that are available to the best advantage. It should allow readers to judiciously interpret the results of such analyses and to do so with methodological rigor or modesty.

This chapter provides some context for the interest shown by epidemiologists, demographers, and social scientists in the analysis of the association of age, period, and cohort to key dependent variables, and draws on examples from several substantive areas. Since the focus involves the same three independent variables (age, period, and cohort), the substantive areas are signaled by the outcome variable used, such as fertility rates, tuberculosis rates, mortality rates, suicide rates, support for same sex marriages, or trust in government.[*]

1.2 Interest in Age, Period, and Cohort

From one perspective, the age–period–cohort (APC) conundrum seems like an esoteric problem that should be of concern only to specialists in quantitative methods. From another perspective this conundrum is at the heart of large bodies of research in demography, economics, epidemiology, political science, sociology, and related areas. This claim may seem contrary to the empirical literature. How often in this literature do we actually read of researchers trying to grapple with age, period, and cohort in their research? Unfortunately, it is not often enough. We often, however, find researchers using age in cross-sectional analysis or shifts in the behavior of young people or the elderly across periods. Researchers also use two of these variables in a single model, such as examining the age distribution of a disease or suicide, or attitudes across a series of periods. In each of these cases the APC identification problem lurks, often unseen, in the background.

1.2.1 Age Alone

What if a researcher finds that the age distribution for lung cancer mortality peaks at age 45 to 54 in a cross-sectional study conducted in 1970? This interesting finding might tell us something about the propensity of certain age groups to die from lung cancer. It might provide clues into the etiology of lung cancer. On its surface, this finding might seem to have nothing to do with the APC problem, but on closer inspection it is intimately linked to that problem. This simple age distribution could easily result from cohort differences in exposure to smoking. Those 45–54 in 1970 are members of the cohort that was age 15–24 in 1940 (an age when the smoking habit is presumably formed). If 1940 was a period in which the recruitment of smokers was at a very high level (more so than cohorts before or after this time), then this cohort when its members were age 45–54 would (all other things being equal) have higher rates of lung cancer mortality than other age groups.

---

[*] Throughout this book the focus is on repeated cross-sectional data rather than panel data in which the same individuals are followed over time. An assumption that is implicit throughout is that the population does not change significantly over time due to migration or other factors that could affect the relationships between the dependent variable and the age, period, and cohort factors.

Examining age alone does not solve the APC problem; it only ignores this potential cohort effect. This cross-sectional age distribution could be a function of age alone, cohort alone, or age and cohort together.

1.2.2 Period Alone

When examining a time series, a researcher may find that for those 30–39 years old there is a trend of increasing support for same sex marriages in national polls and conclude that this shows that over time people are becoming more supportive of the idea of same sex marriage. This period-effect interpretation, implies that people are changing their views over time. But it may be just as likely that this is a cohort effect, with more recent cohorts being more supportive of same sex marriages than previous cohorts. That is, it is not shifts in people's attitudes that drive this change, but the same age group being represented by more recent cohorts in more recent periods: a cohort effect. Again examining periods alone does not solve the APC problem; it simply ignores one explanation for another. Perhaps in this case, the shift in support for same sex marriage is a period effect alone, or a cohort effect alone, or a period and cohort effect together.

1.2.3 Cohort Alone

A much rarer type of analysis examines cohorts alone. One might compare a series of cohorts when they were at the same age (age 40–49) and determine whether there is a relationship in which some cohorts have higher levels of support for social welfare programs in this middle-age voter group. If there appear to be systematic differences between cohorts, is this due to cohort effects or is it due to period effects? The 40–49 age group in each of the cohorts is associated with a different period. These apparent cohort effects could be a function of cohorts alone, of period alone, or of cohort effects and period effects.

In the aforementioned age-alone design, the period effect is controlled by examining age within a single period. For the period-alone design the age effect is controlled by examining a single age group. For the cohort-alone, design described previously, the age effect is controlled by examining a single age group. In each of these cases, the potential for a misspecification is high (the relationship between two variables may be fully or partially dependent on another variable that has been left out of the model). Even when we include two of these variables—age and period, age and cohort, or period and cohort—this threat of misspecification exists. As an example, I begin with the common research design in which the researcher examines the age distribution of some relevant dependent variable such as homicide rates, tuberculosis rates, or support for same sex marriage over time. The question might be whether the age effect is stable over time.

1.2.4 Age–Period Explanation

In criminology the age distributions of homicide offending and several other crimes have been labeled invariant (Hirschi and Gottfredson 1983), but others have challenged this notion (Greenberg 1985; Steffensmeier, Allan, Harer, and Streifel 1989). In the middle 1980s the age distribution of homicide changed dramatically with the rates for those 15–19 years old more than doubling, those for individuals aged 20–24 and 25–29 increasing, while those of all older age groups declined. Is this shift across periods in the propensity of different age groups to commit homicide a shift that we should expect to be the new norm for homicide offending representing a new and stable age effect? Could it be something lasting that is related to period changes, such as shifts in the roles that are assigned to young adults, shifts in criminal justice policies involving young adults, or some other period changes related to the age distribution of homicide offending? Perhaps, however, these shifts in the age distribution across periods could be attributed to cohort effects that in this case are confounded with the age distribution of homicide, since each age is represented by a different cohort during each period. The age distribution at each period is a function of more than age and period, and in the APC context we must consider the potential role of cohorts (O'Brien, Stockard, and Isaacson 1999).

1.2.5 Age–Cohort Explanation

A researcher might use this approach to investigate the effects of age to see whether as people age there are some similarities or differences in the relationship of age to the dependent variable of interest across cohorts. The dependent variable could be an age–cohort-specific score on a political conservatism scale, support for same sex marriage, or the age–cohort-specific cancer mortality rates at different ages. The researcher might find that across several cohorts there is the same pattern of increases with age. If the pattern of age is similar for the different cohorts, this would seem to support the conclusion that a particular age effect is the cause of the pattern. This is certainly a possibility, but the pattern may be due to period effects. This confusion is probably most likely, if there is a linear period effect that is seen as an increase or decrease in the dependent variable with age. But other patterns can be quite confusing. More concretely, if approval for same sex marriage is a period effect with there being a general cultural shift toward support for same sex marriage over time, then this would appear to be an age effect within cohorts with an increasing level of support as the cohort ages. More likely there are age and period effects. Disentangling such effects is part of the APC problem.

1.2.6 Age–Period–Cohort Explanation

Given the potential for confounding when age, period, or cohort are analyzed alone or in pairs, one might expect that formal recognition of the role of all three of these variables in models would be the norm. The norm, however, is to use one or a pair of these variables in analyses. When all three of these variables appear in the same analysis, age, period, and cohort are confounded, because they are linearly dependent. The effects of one of these factors cannot be fully separated from the other two factors. In the simplest case where age, period, and cohort are coded linearly (in years), if we know the period and the age of people in a category, we can determine their birth cohort: Period – Age = Cohort. The question asked might be whether the relationship of cohort to the dependent variable is associated with cohort effects or with the period effects minus the age effects. There is no way to decide except by making an assumption about the relationship between these three variables. This is the focus of this book. We investigate this issue and strategies to gain information from such models when the data that we have is at the aggregate level. This is the level of much data provided by government agencies and the classic focus of APC models.

1.3 Importance of Cohorts

Compared to age groups and periods, which play prominent roles in much social and behavioral science research, cohorts have been *relatively* ignored in the literature.* This tendency also exists in the general public. When mentioning that age plays a role in homicide rates, birth rates, and political conservatism or that there have been shifts in the tuberculosis rates and suicide rates over time, these statements are relatively easy for people to understand. The follow-up question often is about what is or has been the pattern of the age distribution or changes in the age distribution over time. When mentioning that cohorts or birth cohorts play a role in tuberculosis rates or homicide rates, the likely response is the question: What is a cohort? Even after explaining what a cohort is, there is typically some difficulty in conceiving of the association of cohorts with rates of homicide or tuberculosis. People seem less attuned to thinking in terms of cohorts or at least less accustomed to doing so. When cohort differences are presented as generational differences such as baby boom versus baby bust generations, however, understanding comes more easily. To say that the generation that came of age during the Great Depression is more frugal with money or politically more liberal seems to be more understandable to the layperson.

In this chapter I review an admittedly highly selected set of works related in different ways to the general problem of working with age groups, periods,

---

* This is not meant to say that cohorts are ignored by demographers, epidemiologists, and social scientists (far from it), but only that age is a standard variable in much cross-sectional work and periods in time series analysis. Cohorts are less routinely the focus of study.

and cohorts. Several landmark papers exist in different disciplines that serve as touchstones for encouraging the disciplines to increase their focus on cohorts and on the complications that arise from the confounding of the effects of age groups, periods, and cohorts. In demography and sociology, one landmark paper is Norman Ryder's (1965) "The Cohort as a Concept in the Study of Social Change." That paper and both disciplines note the work of Karl Mannheim (1928/1952) in "The Problem of Generations." Mannheim's own work cites Hume and Comte. Neither of these papers focuses on the analysis of empirical data, but instead they are discursive pleas for researchers to focus on cohorts and their role in social change and stability. The Lexis diagram, which dates from the 1860s or 1870s[*] (discussed later in this chapter), does not tout the importance of cohorts, though the Lexis diagram is central in relating time since birth, age, and period. A touchstone paper in epidemiology and one that involves the examination of empirical data was crafted by Wade Hampton Frost (1939) and published shortly after his death in 1938. The life table is central to demography, epidemiology, and actuarial science. In its original development, cohort effects were ignored in the computation of life tables, but cohorts now often play a role in the computation of life tables. We could cite dozens of important precursors to the types of APC models and analyses examined in this book. As noted in the first paragraph of this chapter, however, this book is not about the historical development of the age, period, and cohort analysis. I nonetheless draw on the works just mentioned to provide some sense of the development of an interest in the effects of cohorts in addition to the interest that seems to be more "natural" in the effects age and period.

1.3.1 Life Table

The life table plays a central role in demography and epidemiology (but it also plays a role in criminology, economics, sociology, and other disciplines). John Graunt (1662) is generally considered to have produced the first life table. He notes: "Whereas we have found, that of 100 quick Conceptions about 36 of them die before they be six years old and that perhaps one survived to 76, we, having seven *Decads* between six and 76, we sought six mean proportional numbers between 64, the remainder, living at six years, and the one, which survives 76…" Note that Graunt included only live births (quick conceptions) so the number dying at birth is zero. He also needed to "estimate" the number dying in 10-year periods between the ages of 6 and 76. The result was the data that constitute Table 1.1. This table represents a crude attempt at a life table in part because the *Bills of Mortality* from which Graunt compiled this

---

[*] Though one can question whether this diagram originated with the economist Lexis in 1874 or with Zeuner (1869) or Brasche (1870) as noted in (Vandeschrick 2001), it is associated with the name Lexis.

TABLE 1.1

Crude Life Table of London Constructed
by John Graunt (1662)

Age in Years	Number Dying	Number Surviving
Birth	0	100
6	36	64
16	24	40
26	15	25
36	9	16
46	6	10
56	4	6
66	3	3
76	2	1
86	1	0

Source: Graunt, J., 1662, *Natural and Political Observations upon the Bills of Mortality* (1st edition).
Note: Based on a hypothetical population of 100 live births.

data did not include the age of the deceased (Glass 1950) and the measures used in a modern life table had yet to be invented.

A modern life table indicates much more than Graunt's crude table; for example, the probability of a person dying at a certain age (between two birthdays), the number of people surviving to a certain age (out of 100,000), and the life expectancy for people at different ages. Not surprisingly the data used to construct such tables is much better than the data available to Graunt, as are the methods for estimating the probability of death at age x or the average years of life remaining for members of a cohort still alive at age x (Bell and Miller 2005). In contrast, Graunt estimated, however crudely, the number of people dying between certain ages and the number surviving at particular ages. For example, of those live births, 36 in 100 died by the time they were 6 and thus 64 survived to that age; between the ages of 6 and 16, he estimated that 24 more died and now only 40 of those live births survived at the age of 16. It was a commendable first step. The life table is tremendously important in epidemiology, in demography, in other social sciences, in the insurance industry, and for pension funds. For our purposes, it is intimately related to the problem of separating age, period, and cohort effects.

The easiest form of a life table to construct is the standard *period life table* that is based on the mortality experiences of the entire population in a particular period (a single year or averages across a few consecutive years). This means that when a 20-year-old woman reads a period life table and finds that her life expectancy is 59 years, that expectation is not based on the experience of her cohort. It is based instead on the number of years lived beyond that age by the members of other cohorts, all born earlier than her cohort. We know, for instance, that in the United States the expected length of life at birth for cohorts has increased over time. Therefore, the estimated life expectancy at any age based on the period life table is likely to be an underestimate of the life expectancy of those from more recent cohorts. The 20-year-old woman probably has a life expectancy (years of life remaining) that is greater than 59 years.

Notice how the APC problem relates to the period life table. This table bases estimates of the probability of death at age x (during that year of life) or the life expectancy at age 20 on the mortality experiences of the entire population during a particular period. This ignores the differences in the mortality experiences of cohorts (at least their experiences in the ages they have not yet obtained in the period life table).

Cohort life tables address this problem. Some are based on the mortality experiences of cohorts throughout their life spans, but these tables "do not work" for someone who is 20 and wants to know his life expectancy, since members in his cohort have not yet passed the age of 20, and it does not work for a life insurance company that provides life insurance or the Social Security Administration trying to plan for future beneficiaries. The key insight here is that there is something distinct about cohorts beyond the fact that they age. Other cohort life tables are based on their mortality experiences for past years and projections of future years, and for cohorts not yet born projections into the future alone. Still others are based entirely on projections. These projections can be built into modeling a life table by taking into consideration trends in life spans and work well in a situation in which the increase or decrease in life spans is consistent over a long period of time (for example, see Bongaarts 2005; Denton and Spencer 2011; Lee and Carter 1992).

Life tables are very useful for practical and theoretical reasons, but for our purposes they help to pose some of the problems of age–period–cohort analysis. For example, is the proper way to think about an increase in life span as a cohort phenomenon with the life span increasing for each successive cohort or is it to take a period perspective and think of the life span as increasing in each successive period? What is driving this phenomenon: a period effect in which medicine and environmental conditions improve in successive years; or a cohort effect in which inoculation programs, less exposure to diseases with a long latency periods, and better medical care for the young improves the overall health of successive cohorts? Is it a combination of both period and cohort effects and, if so, what is the importance of the contribution of each of these effects.

1.3.2 Lexis Diagram and the Coding of Cohorts

The Lexis diagram was developed to illustrate population dynamics and to aid in the development of life table formulas. For our purposes, it illustrates the relationship between the year of birth, the age of a person during a specific year, and the period (current year). These years are often aggregated, for example, those born between 1900 and 1904. The Lexis diagram in Figure 1.1

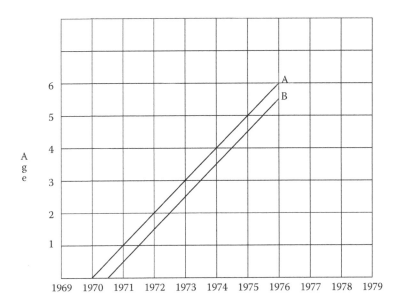

FIGURE 1.1
A Lexis diagram depicting the relationship between year, age, and time since birth.

helps illustrate the complications that arise in determining age, period, and cohort for grouped or ungrouped data. I selected two different times of birth and note the age of the two people in different years. The first person (person A) was born on January 1 of 1970 and the second person (person B) was born in the middle of 1970. On January 1, 1972, person A is 2 years old and remains 2 throughout the 1972 calendar year. But this nice symmetry is not the case for person B. Person B is age 1 for the first half of 1972 and then turns 2 at midyear. She remains 2 through the first half of 1973. For this reason there is not a consistent relationship between year of birth and age. Not all people who were born in 1970 and die in 1980 are 10 years old when they die. Some are 10 years of age and some are 9 years of age.

This creates problems when using archival data that indicate only the age and year of death. For example, homicide offending data from the Federal Bureau of Investigation Uniform Crime Reports or mortality data reported in *Vital Statistics in the United States* provide yearly accounts of the age of the person arrested for homicide or the person who committed the suicide and the year in which the event occurred. This information, however, does not tell us the year in which the person was born and that information is needed to determine their birth cohort. For example, someone who committed homicide in 2000 and was 29 years old could have been born in 1970, but he might have been born in 1971. If he had been born on October 1 of 1970, as long as he murdered someone before that date in 2000 he would be 29 and on or after that date he would be 30. From existing records that record the age of the person committing suicide and the year, we might assume that the person was born in 1970. But he could also have been born in 1971, since someone born on October 1 of 1971 will be 28 before his birthday in 2000 and 29 on or after his birthday in 2000. Knowing the age and year does not determine whether he is a member of the 1970 or the 1971 birth cohort.

Often outcome variables such as the rates of suicide, tuberculosis, or the proportion favoring gay marriage are aggregated into 5-year categories. For example, rates for those age 15–19, 20–24, ..., 75–79. One might then gather data from the National Vital Statistics system of deaths by suicide from 1935, 1940, ..., 2010. This is a nice match of 5-year intervals for the periods with ages aggregated for 5 years. Given this data available from vital statistics, the next question is what are the birth cohorts that correspond to these age–period combinations. Stockard and O'Brien (2002) label (for example) those aged 20–24 in 1980 as belonging to the cohort born between 1955 and 1959, but a different researcher might choose to characterize this cohort as those born between 1956 and 1960, because some of those born in 1960 will be age 20 for part of 1980.

This is not just a question of how the cohort should be labeled, but can have empirical implications for the measurement of key variables. As an example, Stockard and O'Brien (2002) use relative cohort size as a cohort-related variable; that is, it takes the same value for all cases of the same cohort. The measure of relative cohort size they use is based on the percentage of those who are 15 to 64 who are in the cohort when the cohort is 15 to 19. This index compares the relative size of the birth cohort (at a crucial stage for making a shift into adult roles) to the size of the generations preceding it. Not surprisingly the value of relative cohort size will vary depending upon whether we operationalize the cohort as those born between 1955 and 1959 or between 1956 and 1960. Given the 5-year cohorts utilized in this case, the measure is not likely to be much affected.

The aforementioned approach to aggregating the data does not aggregate data across several periods, and it is the one that I have used in my own research. Often researchers aggregate the data for periods. Period data might be based on the average for the dependent variable across each of the age categories for 1930–1934 periods. For example, the age groups might be 5-year age groups 15–19, 20–24, ..., 60–64, and for the youngest age group the dependent variable value would be the average tuberculosis mortality rate for 15–19 year olds for the years 1930 to 1934. The cohorts then have the problem illustrated by the Lexis diagram to an exaggerated degree. Someone who is 15 to 19 in 1930 might be considered to be a member of the cohort that was born as early as 1910 or as late as 1919 (or perhaps 1911 to 1920). This 10-year span for cohorts is created by aggregating the period data. It is why I prefer not aggregating the periods; however, the method I prefer considers only one-fifth of the data on the dependent variable available in this example.

I will not delve into the literature on how to estimate the birth cohort that best corresponds to those of certain ages in a particular period. Some recent developments and citations to the work of others can be found in

Carstensen (2007, 2008) and Rosenbauer and Strassburger (2008). Typically, however, researchers do not attempt to correct for this error assuming that it will make only minor differences in the results of the typical APC analysis, especially when individual ages are grouped into larger age groups. But researchers should carefully consider the data in their particular situation. Corrected or not, the modeling strategies suggested in this book hold as does the linear dependency between age, period, and cohort. That linear dependency (as we will see) depends on a one-to-one relationship between the coding of periods, ages, and cohorts, and all of the examples in this section are examples where a single period–age combination is associated with only one cohort. You will see in the literature and in this book, however, examples of researchers labeling the years associated with cohorts differently for those in the same 5-year age group and the same period.

1.3.3 Frost's Paper

Frost's paper appeared, posthumously, in the *American Journal of Hygiene* in 1939 and was reprinted in the *American Journal of Epidemiology* in 1995. It is considered a classic paper, because it clearly points out that tuberculosis mortality rates in an age–period table might not reflect just age effects and period effects, but might better be viewed as cohort effects (Comstock 2001; Doll 2001). Frost's data for males is presented in an age–period table reformatted as Table 1.2. I have set up the table in the same manner as the Lexis diagram. That is, with age on the vertical axis and the youngest age group being at the bottom of this axis and the oldest age group at the top. Period is

TABLE 1.2

Frost's (1939) Tuberculosis Mortality Rates per 100,000 for Males

Age	1880	1890	1900	1910	1920	1930
70+	672	396	343	163	127	95
60–69	475	340	304	246	172	95
50–59	366	325	267	252	171	*127*
40–49	364	336	253	253	*175*	118
30–39	378	368	296	*253*	164	115
20–29	444	361	*288*	207	149	81
10–19	126	*115*	90	63	49	21
5–9	*43*	49	31	21	24	11
0–4	*760*	578	309	209	108	41

Source: Frost, W.H., 1939, The age selection of mortality from tuberculosis in successive decades, *American Journal of Hygiene* 30:91–96, reprinted from *American Journal of Epidemiology*, 1995, 141:4–9.

Note: The bolded and italicized rates are for the cohort born between 1871 and 1880; Frost labels this cohort the 1880 cohort. The reason for the bolding of two cells in 1880 is that those age groups are both part of the 1880 cohort.

on the horizontal axis with the earliest period at the left and the most recent period at the right. Because of this setup, the cohorts are on the diagonal axis that begins lower on the left and ends higher on the right.*

In his own table Frost bolded and italicized the cell entries that belong to the 1880 cohort (he designated these age groups as born between 1871 and 1880, and labeled them the 1880 cohort). This is the group labeled 0–4 and 5–9 in 1880. Following the earlier discussion, he could have designated this cohort as born between 1870 and 1879. If this table is examined from a period perspective, one sees a dramatic decrease in the rates of tuberculosis. There is almost a perfect monotonic decrease in the rates of tuberculosis for each individual age group across periods. The age distribution for each of the periods exhibits the following pattern: there is a high rate for those 0–4 followed by a dramatic decrease in the 5–9 age group, with an increase until at least middle age. This increase with age pattern is marked for the first three periods where the highest rates (except for the 0–4 category) are for those 70 and older. The relationship is less marked for the most recent three periods with the highest rates being in either the 40–49 or 50–59 age categories (although there is a tie for 1910 between the 30–39 and 40–49 age categories). There seems to be a shift in the age distribution of the rate of mortality due to tuberculosis over these periods, with the youngest age group and the older age groups having the highest rates in the earlier periods and the middle age groups the highest rates in the later periods. Is this a shift in the age-group susceptibility to tuberculosis over time or could differences in cohorts be involved?

Frost points to the interesting relationship found on the diagonals running from lower on the left to higher on the right in the table (the data reflecting the birth cohorts). Here the rates tell a different story (a cohort story). Examining each of the cohorts separately, the rates for the very young (0–4) are high and then drop immediately for the (5–9) age category. For the cohorts that cover enough age groups, the rates then grow to a maximum for the age group 20–29 and drop as the age of cohort members increases. The pattern for women (not reported here) is almost identical. This pattern is remarkably consistent.

Figure 1.2 shows this pattern graphically for the cohorts in Table 1.2 for which we have data that extends through the age group 20–29. Within these cohorts the age curves are remarkably consistent. The rates are high for the very young (0–4), drop to a low rate for those 5–9, increase to age 20–29, and drop thereafter. As emphasized throughout this book, with data involving the factors age, period, and cohort, there are many different ways to explain relationships as combinations of these three factors.

---

* William Mason and Herbert Smith (1985) extended and corrected Frost's data and analyzed it. I have chosen to keep the data in its original form for this graphical presentation. Their conclusions using the extended data are not dissimilar to my own.

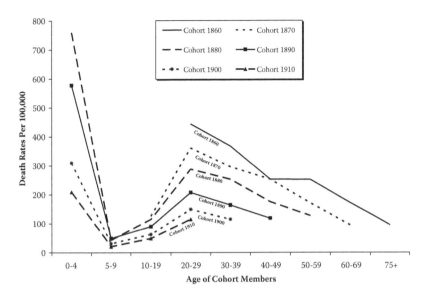

FIGURE 1.2
Within-cohorts age-specific mortality rates from tuberculosis among men in Massachusetts. (Based on Frost, W.H., 1939, The age selection of mortality from tuberculosis in successive decades, *American Journal of Hygiene* 30:91–96.)

This is where theory and past research can play a crucial role. Are there strong reasons, based on theory and on research examining the factors that influence tuberculosis mortality, to expect that the propensity to die from tuberculosis due to age should have shifted over time? If one does not find such evidence, then the consistent age distribution when viewed from the intracohort pattern (see Figure 1.2) provides support for a cohort-based explanation. But for the cohort perspective to be plausible, there must be something about cohorts that makes their propensity to tuberculosis differ and those differences to endure over the life span of the cohort (that is, the approximate pattern in Figure 1.2). We know that tuberculosis is an infectious disease and, during the span of years examined by Frost, it was much more prevalent in the early periods than the more recent ones. When the disease is widespread more people are likely to be infected. In the case of tuberculosis, after a person is infected, the disease often remains latent for years and even decades until there is an opportunity for it to become active.* This, coupled with age differences in proneness to tuberculosis mortality and the public health efforts to eradicate and treat the disease across periods, is certainly compatible with the data displayed in Table 1.2 and Figure 1.2.

---

* It is estimated that about 90% of those infected with TB have asymptomatic (latent) TB infections. Those with asymptomatic, latent TB, have only a 10% lifetime chance that the latent infection will progress to the TB disease (Kumar, Abbas, Fausto, and Mitchell 2007).

1.3.4 Cohorts as Engines of Social Change

As noted earlier, it is obvious to researchers that age is a very important variable. Disease rates, homicide rates, suicide rates, and opinions vary by age. Period is a fundamental variable for disciplines ranging from economics to history. We know that depressions, wars, and empires come and go, and that they affect the behavior of individuals in many ways and many social phenomena such as death rates, and marriage rates, and opinions vary over time. But researchers less often pay attention to cohorts or generations. That is not to say that they are ignored, but only that the relationship of age or year (period) to these phenomena are more often analyzed than is the relationship of cohort to these same phenomena.*

In this section I discuss two classic arguments for the importance of cohorts in the process of social change: Mannheim (1928/1952) and Ryder (1965). But the consideration of cohorts as key elements of change did not originate with them (though they deserve credit for clearly delineating the importance of cohorts). Central to the conception of cohorts as promoters of social change is the idea that certain events (baby booms and baby busts or coming of age in the Great Depression) have an enduring effect on the members of a cohort. That does not mean that the effect may not wane somewhat or wax somewhat, but it often tends to persist. It most decidedly does not mean that all members of the cohort are affected in the same manner, but only that different cohorts have different propensities to generate tuberculosis deaths, suicides, or support of gay marriage.

Karl Mannheim in his classic chapter (1928/1952) first notes some of the previous philosophical conjectures on the role of cohorts in producing stability and change in human societies. He acknowledges Hume for an early discussion of how cohorts provide continuity in human populations: human populations are not like some insect populations that all die out in the spring and then have an entirely new generation. That is, new cohorts do not replace the entire population, but only part of the population. That provides the opportunity for socialization—the passing on of culture and ways of behaving. Socialization and the rigid transmission of culture are not perfect, and cohorts differ from one another in their behaviors and values. Mannheim credits Comte with the following view: "If the average span of life of every individual were either shortened or lengthened, he said, the tempo of progress would also change. This is because the go slow conservative attitudes of the older generation would not be so strong in short generations" (p. 277). Mannheim died before the middle of the 20th century and in that sense he should perhaps not be considered a "modern figure" in the development

---

* I am trying to be careful in this statement. It is an empirical fact that researchers more often use age and period (time) in their analyses than they use cohorts. That is not to say that cohort are ignored or that they are not the subject of much research and theorizing in epidemiology, demography, and the social sciences.

of thinking about cohorts, but he clearly conceived of their importance as agents of social change.

Norman Ryder is for demographers and sociologists the person who probably first comes to mind when they think about cohorts. In his classic article (1965:843), he notes the work of Mannheim and discusses what he labels *demographic metabolism*: "Society persists despite the mortality of its individual members, through processes of demographic metabolism and particularly the annual infusion of birth cohorts. These may pose a threat to stability, but they also provide the opportunity for societal transformation." Humorously, he labels the appearance of a new cohort "the invasion of barbarians." This is telling metaphor for the problem of socialization faced by both the younger cohorts and their parental generation; it also reflects the possibility of change or differences between cohorts. Ryder emphasizes a point that is at the core of the approach taken in this book, an interest in aggregates: "Changes in an individual throughout his life are distinguishable from changes in the population of which he is a component" (p. 843).

1.3.5 Concluding Remarks

In this section I have emphasized the importance of cohorts. I am not advocating for the dominance of this particular effect over the effects of age or period. Cohorts are highlighted instead because they are often the left out factor in the age, period, and cohort triad. At times it may be appropriate to highlight one of these three factors for special treatment. Age effects can at times be *relatively fixed* for biological reasons, and at other times age effects may shift due to the relationship between age and important life course events, such as changes in marriage rates, fertility rates, and shifts in Social Security or the retirement age. Period effects can also be dramatic: the impact of wars, depressions, or new medical discoveries. Certainly the variance in the effects of variables across period, cohorts, and age groups play a major role. A small change in relative cohort size is not likely to make much of a difference in its impact on a dependent variable. Similarly, small differences in unemployment rates across periods are not likely to have much of an effect. On the other hand, a depression will affect many outcome variables during a particular period, and a baby boom or baby bust may have major effects on cohorts across extended spans of time.

1.4 Plan for the Book

Deciding what topics to cover in this book required many choices, since the literature on APC modeling is immense. One major decision was to limit coverage to aggregate-level data. Aggregate-level data is the form in which most government/official data is published and available in archives; for example, the Uniform Crime Reports and Vital Statistics. It is on this aggregate level that most of the literature on APC models has focused.[*] Another major decision was to recognize that a book-length treatment is appropriate only as an introduction to APC models and analysis. This is such a treatment; it is written for those with a quantitative/statistical background that ideally includes a familiarity with matrix algebra and linear geometry. There certainly are aggregate-level techniques that are not covered, for example, smoothing and Bayesian techniques (Fu 2008; Nakamura 1986), the cohort replacement approach of Firebaugh (1989) that considers the total changes due to cohort replacement and not just cohort-specific change, and special parameterizations of the APC model (Carstensen 2007). The focus is on models that incorporate (in some ways) the effects of all three of factors: age, period, and cohort.

This introductory chapter provides an intuitive introduction to the linear dependency problem and shows why researchers are interested in the separate effects of age controlling for period and cohort, the effects of period controlling for age and cohort, and the effects of cohort controlling for period and age. The confounding effects of linear dependency were illustrated by discussing models that use age alone, period alone, cohort alone, and models that use just two of these factors. In each of those cases, the effects can be due to the omitted factor or factors. A few important pieces of work in the literature were then discussed to shed light on and demonstrate the importance of the APC perspective: life tables, the Lexis diagram, Frost's examination of tuberculosis data, and Mannheim and Ryder's discussion of the importance of cohorts.

Chapter 2 examines what might be labeled the beginning of the modern statistical approach to the APC problem that includes all three of these factors in a single model and uses constrained estimation to find a solution. Unfortunately there is an infinite number of solutions due to the linear dependency between age, period, and cohort. Because the estimates of the individual effect coefficients in the APC model depend upon the constraint used, there needs to be a credible reason for selecting a particular constraint. Despite the problem of justifying the constraint used, such models provide some useful information about the solution. For example, each of the constrained solutions is a least squares solution. Each of the constrained solutions lies on the same line in multidimensional space, and the constrained solutions can be viewed as "rotations" of one another. These sorts of

---

[*] The literature contains work that considers age, period, and cohort at the individual level, where, for example, birth cohort may be used as a contextual variable (Alwin 1991; Wilson and Gove 1999). There also are mixed modeling analyses as suggested by (Yang and Land 2006). I do not investigate methods that depend on panel data that follow individuals over time.

relationships are exploited in the strategies described in later chapters. They help to provide researchers with information about the relationships of age, period, and cohort, and the interpretation of those relationships. I provide an example of the plausible use of constrained estimation. The depiction of the APC model in this chapter depends mainly on matrix algebra.

Chapter 3 focuses on the geometry underlying the underidentification of the APC model. First, I show geometrically that all of the infinite number of least squares solutions lie on a single "line of solutions" in multidimensional space. I then show how constrained solutions force the hyperplane that does not intersect the line of solutions to be reoriented to intersect the line of solutions at a point and thus provide a solution to the APC model under a specified constraint. Chapter 3 reinforces and extends our conception of what a constrained solution is and how it is obtained. It is perhaps the most novel chapter in the book and, for that reason, the approach taken may be difficult for some readers.* The line of solutions discussed in Chapters 2 and 3 plays a prominent role in Chapter 4.

Chapter 4 introduces estimable functions. Although the individual age group, period, and cohort parameter estimates in the APC model cannot be solved uniquely (in terms of providing estimates of the parameters that generated the outcome values), they can be used to provide solutions to certain functions of these parameters. For example, they can be used to determine the deviation of the period effects from the linear trend in the period effects or to find the second differences of the age effects: $(a_3 - a_2) - (a_2 - a_1) = a_1 - 2a_2 + a_3$. These functions of the period effects and the age effects are the same no matter which constraint is used to identify the APC model. The derivations of estimable functions in the literature have used a variety of different methods. Chapter 4 provides a unified derivation of these estimable functions based on the line of solutions. These estimable functions are put to work showing how they can be used with substantive data.

Chapter 5 introduces the variance decomposition of an APC model. Although the age, period, and cohort effect coefficients that generated the outcome values cannot be identified, the unique variance in the outcome variable that is associated with each of these factors can be identified: the variance uniquely associated with the age effects, the variance uniquely associated with the period effects, and the variance uniquely associated with the cohort effects. This provides a sufficient, but not necessary, condition for the existence of statistically significant age effects, period effects, and cohort effects. Several models of variance decomposition are discussed: the APC ANOVA approach (O'Brien and Stockard 2009), the APC mixed model approach (O'Brien, Hudson,

---

* Chapter 3 could be skipped and the remaining chapters would still be understandable. The chapter, however, provides an enhanced sense of the problem that is at the heart of the APC conundrum: structural underidentification.

and Stockard 2008), and (venturing slightly outside of the expressed boundaries of the book) the hierarchical APC approach of Yang and Land (2006) that involves both aggregated and individual-level data. These approaches provide some useful information, but I also discuss their limitations.

Chapter 6 discusses a strategy for identifying APC models that uses characteristics associated with age groups, periods, and cohorts rather than the categorical variables for age or for period or for cohort. Rather than coding cohorts using dummy variable coding a researcher might code some characteristic of cohorts that plausibly accounts for the cohort effects (or part of the cohort effects). For example, a cohort characteristic could be the mean number of years before age 35 that members of a birth cohort were cigarette smokers. Since one *cannot* determine the mean number of years smoking of each of the cohorts by knowing the age and period alone, this breaks the linear dependency: Period – Age ≠ Mean number of years smoking. The advantages and disadvantages of using this and similar approaches are discussed, and some examples of the information provided by these factor characteristics using suicide data as the outcome variable are presented.

The concluding chapter, Chapter 7, focuses on a single empirical example to show how the approaches discussed in this book can be used to provide a credible analysis of the relationships of ages, periods, and cohorts to a dependent variable. The analysis begins by showing what we know to be true (given that the full APC model is the correct specification) based on estimable functions/variance decomposition. To move beyond these "certainties," I emphasize the need for using substantive knowledge and theory when working with APC analyses. Thus, I analyze data in my own substantive area—an analysis of trends in the homicide rates by age and over time—and use both constrained regression and factor characteristic approaches. The findings gain strength from the consistency of the results across several of these approaches.

This book concentrates on creating a unified presentation: showing the APC linear dependency problem algebraically (Chapter 2) and the same problem using a geometrical representation (Chapter 3). A key finding from both of these chapters is that the best fitting solutions to the constrained APC models all lie on the same line in multidimensional space. This provides a key to establishing estimable functions in Chapter 4 as well as the variance decomposition in Chapter 5. The linear dependency motivates the use factor characteristics for age groups and/or periods and/or cohorts in Chapter 6. The interpretation of the results from the factor-characteristic approach relies on insights gained in the previous chapters. Integrating these approaches in one book and emphasizing both the geometry and algebra of several APC approaches, puts the researcher in a stronger position when judging the strengths and weaknesses of these methods. This should facilitate better research and better interpretation and evaluation of existing research.

References

Alwin, D. 1991. Family of origin and cohort differences in verbal ability. *American Sociological Review* 56:625–38.

Bell, F.C., and M.L. Miller. 2005. *Life Tables for the United States Social Security Area 1900–2100* (Actuarial Study number 120). Washington D.C.: Social Security Administration.

Bongaarts, J. 2005. Long-range trends in adult mortality: Models and projection methods. *Demography* 42:23–49.

Brasche, O. 1870. *Beitrag zur Methode der Sterblichkeitsberechnung und Mortalitätsstatistic Bussland's*. Würzburg: A Struber's Buchhandlung.

Cartensen, B. 2007. Age-period-cohort models for the Lexis diagram. *Statistics in Medicine* 26:3018–45.

Cartensen, B. 2008. Author's reply: Age-period-cohort models for the Lexis diagram. *Statistics in Medicine* 27:1561–64.

Comstock, G.W. 2001. Cohort analysis: W.H. Frost's contributions to the epidemiology of tuberculosis and chronic disease. *Social and Preventative Medicine* 46:7–12.

Denton, F.T., and B.G. Spencer. 2011. A dynamic extension of the period life table. *Demographic Research* 24:831–54.

Doll, R. (Sir). 2001. Cohort studies: History of the method 1. Retrospective cohort studies. *Social and Preventative Medicine* 46:152–60.

Firebaugh, G. 1989. Methods for estimating cohort replacement effects. *Sociological Methodology* 19:243–62.

Frost, W.H. 1939. The age selection of mortality from tuberculosis in successive decades. *American Journal of Hygiene* 30:91–96. Reprinted in *American Journal of Epidemiology*, 1995, 141:4–9.

Fu, W.J. 2008. A smoothing cohort model in age-period-cohort analysis with applications to homicide rates and lung cancer mortality rates. *Sociological Methods & Research* 36: 327–61.

Glass, D.V. 1950. Graunt's life table. *Journal of the Institute of Actuaries* 76:60–64.

Graunt, J. 1662. *Natural and Political Observations upon the Bills of Mortality* (1st edition). Available at http://www.edstephan.org/Graunt/bills.html

Greenberg, D. 1985. Age, crime, and social explanation. *American Journal of Sociology*, 91:121.

Hardy, A., and M.E. Magnello. 2004. Statistical methods in epidemiology: Karl Pearson, Ronald Ross, Major Greenwood, and Austin Bradford Hill, 1900–1945. In *A History of Epidemiological Methods and Concepts*, ed. A. Morabia, 205–21. Basel, Switzerland: Birkhäuser Verlag.

Hirschi, T., and M. Gottfredson. 1983. Age and the explanation of crime. *American Journal of Sociology* 89:552–84.

Kumar, V., K.V. Abbas, A.K. Fausto, and R.N. Mitchell (eds.). 2007. *Robbins Basic Pathology* (8th edition). Philadelphia: Saunders Elsevier.

Lee, R.D., and L.R Carter. 1992. Modeling and forecasting U.S. mortality. *Journal of the American Statistical Association* 87:659–71.

Mannheim, K. 1928/1952. The problem of generations. In *Essays on the Sociology of Knowledge*, ed. K. Mannheim (translated and ed. P. Kecskemeti), 276–320. London: Routledge and Kegan Paul.

Mason, W.M., and H.L. Smith. 1985. Age-period-cohort analysis and the study of deaths from pulmonary tuberculosis. In *Cohort Analysis in Social Research: Beyond the Identification Problem*, ed. W.M. Mason and S.E. Fienberg, 151–228. New York: Springer-Verlag.

Nakamura, T. 1986. Bayesian cohort models for general cohort table analysis. *Annals of the Institute of Statistical Mathematics* 38(part B):353–70.

O'Brien, R.M., K. Hudson, and J. Stockard. 2008. A mixed model estimation of age, period, and cohort effects. *Sociological Methods & Research* 36:302–28.

O'Brien, R.M., and J. Stockard. 2009. Can cohort replacement explain changes in the relationship between age and homicide offending? *Journal of Quantitative Criminology* 25:79–101.

O'Brien, R.M., J. Stockard, and L. Isaacson. 1999. The enduring effects of cohort characteristics on age-specific homicide rates, 1960-1995. *American Journal of Sociology* 104:1061–95.

Rosenbauer, J., and K. Strassburger. 2008. Comments on "Age-period-cohort models for the Lexis diagram." *Statistics in Medicine* 27:1557–61.

Ryder, N.B. 1965. The cohort as a concept in the study of social change. *American Sociological Review* 30:843–61.

Steffensmeier, D., E. Allan, M. Harer, and C. Streifel. 1989. Age and the distribution of crime. *American Journal of Sociology* 94:803–31.

Stockard, J., and R.M. O'Brien. 2002. Cohort effects on suicide rates: International variations. *American Sociological Review* 67:854–72.

Vandeschrick, C. 2001. The Lexis diagram, a misnomer. *Demographic Research* 4:97–124.

Wilson, J.A., and W.R. Gove. 1999. The intercohort decline in verbal ability: Does it exist? *American Sociological Review* 64:253–66.

Yang, Y., and K.C. Land. 2006. A mixed models approach to the age-period-cohort analysis of repeated cross-section surveys with an application to data on trends in verbal test scores. *Sociological Methodology* 36:75–97.

Zeuner, G. 1869. Zur mathematischen statistick. *Beilage zur zeitschrift des königlisch sächsischen statistischen bureau*, XXX1 Jahrgang: 1–13.

2

Multiple Classification Models and Constrained Regression

> [M]eaningful three-way cohort analysis is difficult unless the researcher entertains relatively strong hypotheses about the nature of aging, period, and cohort effects.
>
> **K.O. Mason, W.M. Mason, H.H. Winsborough, and W.K. Poole (1973:242)**

2.1 Introduction

The previous chapter indicated some problems with examining only the age distribution, or differences between periods, or differences between cohorts. Many researchers examine two of these variables at a time; for example, an age-by-period table so that they can study how the age distribution of a disease or crime or attitude varies over time. But the shifts in the age distributions across periods can be affected by cohorts. This suggests examining all three of these factors in an age–period–cohort (APC) model. This explicitly raises a new problem: the identification problem that motivated the opening quotation in the article by Mason, Mason, Winsborough, and Poole (1973).

The classic APC problem involves the inability to uniquely estimate the effects of each of the components (age, period, and cohort) separately using a standard regression model. This problem for APC models had its first modern presentation in Mason et al. (1973). Not only did they clearly describe the problem, but they noted that a single constraint would just identify the model. Two other works by Mason and Fienberg (Fienberg and Mason 1979; Mason and Fienberg 1985) helped establish their general approach. Since that time constrained regression has been a much used "solution" to the identification problem.[*] The easiest situation to conceptualize is one that involves a *linear coding* of these factors: for example, coding period as the year of the occurrence, cohort by year of birth, and age in years of age. If the data were

---

[*] They were aware that one could not differentiate the different constrained solutions from one another on the basis of model fit and that the coefficient estimates from the different constraints used in the constrained regression approach could differ greatly.

not available for single years (for example, it was reported in 5-year classes) a researcher still might use linear coding by coding the mean of the periods, the mean birth year, and the mean age. With such coding there is one variable for period, one for cohort, and one for age. If we do not transform any of the variables, this coding limits the form of the relationships between each of the independent variables (age, period, and cohort) and the dependent variable to a linear relationship, but it does not help with the problem of identification.

Even if data are available in single-year categories, researchers may decide that it is best to categorize them into groups of ages and periods and cohorts. Researchers then often code the data categorically: *categorical coding*. For example, the researcher may use categories of age such as those who were 15–19, 20–24, ..., 75–79 who died of tuberculosis and collect this data in the years (periods) 1930, 1935, ..., 2010. The 5-year cohorts corresponding to this categorical coding are 1850–1854, 1865–1869, ..., 1990–1994. In this form, it is typical to treat each of the age groups, periods, and cohorts as different variables (for example, using dummy variable or effect coding) with one category for age groups, one for periods, and one for cohorts reserved as the "reference" category.

2.2 Linearly Coded Age–Period–Cohort (APC) Model

The linear model is briefly discussed because it is simpler to understand than the categorical or multiple-classification model; yet most researchers use the categorical model. Table 2.1 shows schematically the sort of data that might be obtained from a vital statistics program containing yearly data (although this is clearly artificial data). The first row shows 7 cases of tuberculosis death per 100,000 for those aged 41 in the year 2005. We designate these cases as the group of people who were born in 1964 (2005 – 41 = 1964).* Table 2.1 makes clear the linear dependency between age, period, and cohort: Period – Age = Cohort. This linear dependency is evident in all of the rows of the Table 2.1 (whether we examine the original data on the left-hand side of the table or the data in deviation score form on the right-hand side).

Table 2.2 displays this same data in tabular form. Often such tables have the youngest age group in the first row and the oldest in the last row, but for this table I mimic the format of the Lexis diagram from the previous chapter. The table has four ages represented in the rows of the table, four periods

---

* As noted in Chapter 1, when discussing the Lexis diagram some of these people may have been born in 1963 and some of those born in 1964 will be not have reach the age of 41 when they die 2005. This does not change the linear dependency implied by Period – Age – Cohort. After all, this is how we assigned the corresponding cohorts to the ages in the periods.

TABLE 2.1

Illustrative (Author Constructed) Data with Four Ages and Four Periods

	Original Data				Deviation Data			
Intercept	Age	Period	Cohort	y	Age	Period	Cohort	y
1	41	2005	1964	7	−1.5	−1.5	0	−4.5
1	42	2005	1963	6	−0.5	−1.5	−1	−5.5
1	43	2005	1962	5	0.5	−1.5	−2	−6.5
1	44	2005	1961	4	1.5	−1.5	−3	−7.5
1	41	2006	1965	11	−1.5	−0.5	1	−0.5
1	42	2006	1964	10	−0.5	−0.5	0	−1.5
1	43	2006	1963	9	0.5	−0.5	−1	−2.5
1	44	2006	1962	8	1.5	−0.5	−2	−3.5
1	41	2007	1966	15	−1.5	0.5	2	3.5
1	42	2007	1965	14	−0.5	0.5	1	2.5
1	43	2007	1964	13	0.5	0.5	0	1.5
1	44	2007	1963	12	1.5	0.5	−1	0.5
1	41	2008	1967	19	−1.5	1.5	3	7.5
1	42	2008	1966	18	−0.5	1.5	2	6.5
1	43	2008	1965	17	0.5	1.5	1	5.5
1	44	2008	1964	16	1.5	1.5	0	4.5

Note: The y variable is the tuberculosis rate per 100,000.

TABLE 2.2

Data from Table 2.1 Placed in a 4 × 4 Age–Period Table
(Tuberculosis Rates per 100,000 in Parentheses)

	Period			
Age	2005	2006	2007	2008
44	1961 (4)	1962 (8)	1963 (12)	1964 (16)
43	1962 (5)	1963 (9)	1964 (13)	1965 (17)
42	1963 (6)	1964 (10)	1965 (14)	1966 (18)
41	1964 (7)	1965 (11)	1966 (15)	1967 (19)

represented in the columns of the table, and the seven cohorts occupying the diagonals (running from lower left-hand side to upper right-hand side). For example, the cohort born in 1964 has four observations (at age 41 in 2005, age 42 in 2006, age 43 in 2007, and at age 44 in 2008). This diagonal runs from the lower left of the table to the upper right. The cohorts born in 1963 and 1965 have only three observations each, and those born in 1961 and 1967 have only a single observation. The age–period-specific dependent variable values (tuberculosis deaths per 100,000) are in the corresponding cells of this table within parentheses.

Although the analysis of linearly coded age, period, and cohort models will not be pursued, if it were, the data in Table 2.1 or Table 2.2 would be used to run a regression analysis with the tuberculosis rates as the dependent variable and the age, period, and cohort variables as the independent variables.[*] The same problems found in the next several sections of this chapter would be encountered: there is a linear dependency between the three independent variables, there is a linear combination of the columns of the matrix (the intercept and the three independent variables) that makes the sum of each row equal zero; placing a single constraint on the coefficients of the model produces the best fitting solution; these best fitting solutions lie on a line; there are an infinite number of these best fitting solutions; and so on. These topics are now covered in depth in the context of the most frequently used form of APC models: those that use categorical coding. (The linear coding situation is covered in some depth in Chapter 3, where I take advantage of the smaller number of dimensions in the linear model to introduce the geometry of the APC model.)

2.3 Categorically Coded APC Model

Categorical coding of the APC model allows the relationship between the dependent variable and the age groups, periods, and cohorts to take on a wide variety of functional forms; for example, it does not constrain the relationship between age and the dependent variable to be linear or quadratic. Categorical coding allows each category of age, period, and cohort to have its own effect that may be higher or lower than other age groups, periods, or cohorts. I use the following representation for the categorical APC model (here it is based on a rectangular age–period table):

$$Y_{ij} = \mu + \alpha_i + \pi_j + \chi_{I-i+j} + \epsilon_{ij}. \tag{2.1}$$

Y_{ij} is the dependent variable value for the ijth cell of the age–period table; μ is the value of the intercept; α_i is the age effect of the ith age-group; π_j is the period effect for the jth period; χ_{I-i+j} is the cohort effect for the $(I - i + j)$th cohort (where I is the number of age groups), and ϵ_{ij} is the error term or residual associated with the ijth cell of the age–period table. Since age, period, and cohort are categorically coded, one of the age groups, one of the periods, and one of the cohorts serve as reference groups.

The model in matrix notation is written as

$$y = Xb + \epsilon. \tag{2.2}$$

---

[*] Poisson regression and negative binomial regression are other possibilities, but in those cases we would need to know the number of people in each of the age–period groups and the number of deaths due to tuberculosis.

When using categorical coding, X is often labeled the design matrix. It is used to code the intercept and each of the age groups, periods, and cohorts, except those serving as reference categories. Schematically, we can write the columns of the X-matrix as intercept, age_1 to age_{I-1}, $period_1$ to $period_{J-1}$, $cohort_1$ to $cohort_{I+J-2}$, where I is the number of age groups, J is the number of periods, and $I + J - 1$ is the number of cohorts. The number of columns in X is $m = 2(I + J) - 3 = 1 + (I - 1) + (J - 1) + (I + J - 2)$ and the number of rows is $I \times J$. The intercept and the age, period, and cohort categories are in the columns and the rows correspond to the cells of the age–period table. The categorical age, period, and cohort variables are coded in different ways: the two most common approaches are dummy variable coding and effect coding. The outcome vector, y, has as many rows as there are cells in the age–period table, b represents the solution vector with $2(I + J) - 3$ rows, and ϵ is a vector of residuals that has $I \times J$ elements. It is assumed that $E(X'\epsilon) = \mathbf{0}$.[*]

Premultiplying both sides of Equation (2.2) by the transpose of X yields $X'y = X'Xb + X'\epsilon$. Since $E(X'\epsilon) = \mathbf{0}$, the normal equations are typically written as

$$X'Xb = X'y. \tag{2.3}$$

These are the same equations derived by using partial differentiation to find the solutions (b) that minimize the sum of the squared residuals between the predicted and observed values of y. Solving these equations produces least squares solutions.

For the moment, the standard procedure for solving Equation (2.3) are followed, even though we will soon note that this procedure cannot be followed in APC analysis because X is not of full column rank. The next step in the standard procedure is to premultiply both sides of Equation (2.3) by the inverse of $X'X$: $(X'X)^{-1}$. The result is

$$b = (X'X)^{-1} X'y. \tag{2.4}$$

If X were of full column rank Equation (2.4) would provide a unique solution. Assuming that the model is correctly specified, it would provide unbiased estimates of the parameters that generated the y-vector values. Following Greene (1993) our interest is in the estimation of the parameter vector β, in the model $y = X\beta + \epsilon$. This model describes how the y values are "generated" by the parameter values in the vector β and the random error term. When X is of full column rank the solution vector b is an unbiased estimate of the parameter-vector β that generated the y values.[†]

---

[*] The bolded zero represents a vector of zeros.
[†] Remembering that the underlying model that we wish to estimate is $y = X\beta + \epsilon$ and using a bit of algebraic manipulation of the preceding formulas, Greene (993:182) shows that $b = (X'X)^{-1} X' (X\beta + \epsilon) = \beta + (X'X)^{-1} X'\epsilon$ and if $E(X'\epsilon) = 0$, then $E(b) = \beta$. This unbiasedness holds for both nonstochastic and stochastic regressors, although the proofs vary somewhat.

Unfortunately, in the traditional multiple-classification APC model there is a linear dependency among the age, period, and cohort categorical variables—a problem alluded to in the previous chapter. One manifestation of this problem is that the regular inverse $(X'X)^{-1}$ does not exist. This absence of a regular inverse prevents the use of the standard method to solve the normal equations for b as in Equation (2.4). Some packaged programs at this point note that the inverse does not exist, while others drop one of the independent variables and produce *a* least squares solution to the normal equations. Dropping a variable is a warning sign that determining a unique best fitting solution is not possible. The program runs after dropping a variable, because there is not a linear dependency between the age, period, and cohort variables after one of the categorical variables is dropped. By dropping one of the variables, the program assumes that the dropped variable effect is equal to zero. It places a constraint on the model, and this identifies the model. The identification problem in this case is not that there is no solution, but instead that there is an infinite number of solutions to the normal equations (2.3). Depending on which variable is dropped by the program, the solutions will be different in terms of the parameters estimates for the individual coefficients.

This is the APC conundrum (O'Brien 2000). The researcher assumes that the model in Equation (2.2) is the correct specification and wants to know the effects of each of the age, period, and cohort coefficients. These parameters cannot be uniquely estimated without placing a constraint on one or more coefficients in the model. The constraint placed on the coefficients, however, determines which one of the infinite number of solutions for b the analysis provides.

With dummy variable coding each row of X contains a 1 in the first column. For the remaining columns (remembering that each row represents a cell of the age–period table) each row of X contains a 1 in the columns corresponding to the cell represented by the row. If the cell is for the youngest age group in the first period and that corresponds to the fourth cohort, then the columns representing this age group, this period, and this cohort will have a 1 in that particular row. If the row represents a cell that is used as a reference category on age and/or period and/or cohort, it contains zeros in the columns representing that factor. All rows of the table are coded in a similar fashion. All of the other entries in each of the rows are coded with zeros.

Effect coding uses the same procedure for assigning ones to the column elements in each row. The difference is that any row that represents a cell in the reference category for a factor (age and/or period and/or cohort) has minus 1 for the columns representing that factor. For example, suppose that a particular row represents a cell in the reference category for age, then for that row the elements in the age columns are all coded with minus 1. All of the row elements that are not coded with one, or minus one, are coded with a zero. To make this extended verbal description clearer, these two forms of coding using the design matrix for a 4×4 age–period table appear in

Appendix 2.1. Note that there are 16 [= ($I \times J$) = 4 × 4] rows and that there is one column for the intercept, $I - 1$ columns for the age groups, $J - 1$ columns for the periods, and $I + J - 2$ columns for the cohorts.

The problem with Equation (2.4) is that no matter which form of coding is used the inverse $(X'X)^{-1}$ does not exist. $X'X$ is rank deficient by 1, because of the linear dependency between the column variables of X. A solution to the normal equations can be found, however, by using a generalized inverse. The generalized inverse is symbolized as $(X'X)^{-}$ and the solution to the normal equations that it produces can be written as

$$b_c^0 = (X'X)^{-} X'y. \tag{2.5}$$

Here the superscripted negative sign indicates that $(X'X)^{-}$ is a generalized inverse of $X'X$; b_c^0 is *a* solution to the normal equations under a just identifying constraint that is associated with the generalized inverse. Since this is *a* solution to the normal equations, it is *a* least squares solutions. Unfortunately, it is not the only solution to the normal equations; there is an infinite number of solutions each using a different generalized inverse and each being a least squares solution. This means that each of the solutions generates the same set of predicted values ($\hat{y}$) and these different solutions fit the observed data just as well as any other least squares solution. Each solution minimizes the sum of the squared residuals. There are several sources that describe how to construct generalized inverses (e.g., Scheffé 1959; Searle 1971). One source, however, is particularly useful for our purpose (Mazumdar, Li, and Bryce 1980).

Mazumdar, Li, and Bryce (1980) provide a convenient method for creating a generalized inverse that incorporates a particular constraint. Their procedure is simple:

1. Compute $X'X$.
2. Replace the last row of $X'X$ with the constraint. For example, if we wish to constrain the age1 effect to equal the age2 effect with data from a 4 × 4 age–period matrix, we set the following constraint: [(0 × μ) + (1 × a_1) + (–1 × a_2) + (0 × a_3) + ⋯ + (0 × c_6) = 0)]. The vector associated with this constraint is c_1 = (0, 1, –1, 0 ⋯, 0)′, and the last row of $X'X$ is replaced with (0, 1, –1, 0, ⋯, 0).
3. Compute the inverse of this new matrix.
4. Replace the last column of this inverse with a column of zeros.[*] The result is the generalized inverse $(X'X)_{c1}^{-}$ associated with the particular constraint (constraint 1), which when used in Equation (2.5) produces the solution (b_{c1}^0) associated with this constraint.

---

[*] Mazumdar, Li, and Bryce (1980) note that if the constraint is placed in the *i*th row of the $X'X$-matrix, then after obtaining the inverse of this modified matrix, the *i*th column of the inverse of the modified matrix would be replaced with zeros.

Basically this procedure eliminates the linear dependency by removing one of the rows and replacing it (in general) with a row that is not linearly dependent on the other rows. I use the term "in general" because one could replace a row with a constraint that is linearly dependent on the other rows (most likely inadvertently, since the constraint is usually instituted to remove the linear dependency).

There is something distinctive that the solutions to a rank deficient by one set of normal equations share in common. The solutions all lie on a line (in multidimensional space). Why this is the case is demonstrated next.

We could find a solution to the normal equations with a generalized inverse based on a constraint using the Mazumdar, Li, and Bryce (1980) approach, or we could use a constrained regression program, or we could use any appropriate generalized inverse. If b_{c1}^0 is one of these solutions to the normal equations, then

$$X'Xb_{c1}^0 = X'y. \tag{2.6}$$

That is, postmultiplying $X'X$ by b_{c1}^0 produces $X'y$, since b_{c1}^0 is *a* solution to the normal equations. The linear dependency in the APC model occurs because there is a linear combination of the columns of the design matrix, X, that produces a zero vector. That is, $Xv = \mathbf{0}$, where v is labeled the null vector and the bolded zero represents a column vector of zeros. The null vector, v, is unique up to multiplication by a scalar; so we can write $Xsv = \mathbf{0}$, where s is a scalar. There is only one null vector for the APC model, because X is only rank deficient by one in the APC situation.[*] $Xsv = \mathbf{0}$ implies that $X'Xsv = \mathbf{0}$, so we can write,

$$X'y = X'Xb_{c1}^0 + X'Xsv, \tag{2.7}$$

which produces the same values of $X'y$ as (2.6). Rearranging terms in Equation (2.7), note that

$$X'y = X'X(b_{c1}^0 + sv). \tag{2.8}$$

Therefore, if b_{c1}^0 is a solution to the normal equations, and so is $b_{c1}^0 + sv$.

The term in parentheses in Equation (2.8) is the right-hand side of the vector equation for a line in multidimensional space. The vector equation for this line can be written as

$$b_c^0 = b_{c1}^0 + sv. \tag{2.9}$$

---

[*] The "trivial" null vector is typically not counted; it is a vector of all zeros with as many elements as there are columns in X. This vector will always produce a vector of zeros: $Xv = \mathbf{0}$ for any X. The trivial null vector would not change the original solution (b_{c1}^0). If X were rank deficient by two, there would be two nontrivial null vectors and the null space would be of two dimensions.

This line is established by finding one point on the line (for example, b_{c1}^0) and the direction of the line. A solution to the normal equations is a point on the line in multidimensional solution space and v (the null vector) is a direction of the line in multidimensional space. Any solution $\left(b_c^0\right)$ on the line of solutions is a solution to the normal equations.

To establish that the only solutions to the normal equations lie on this line, we note that the design matrix for the APC model (X) is rank deficient by one; therefore, there is only one null vector v (which is unique up to multiplication by a scalar). There is no other sv that can postmultiply $X'X$ and result in the zero vector (except the "trivial vector" consisting of all zeros). Thus, there is one and only one line of solutions for the normal equations.

Note how different the APC situation is from the typical regression situation in which X is of full column rank. In the full column rank situation the model is identified so that there is a unique solution. Using the language of maximum likelihood, that unique solution has the greatest likelihood of having generated outcome data. If the APC model were identified, we would obtain the age, period, and cohort coefficients that were most likely to have generated the outcome variable values given the specification of the model. In the rank deficient by one case, there are an infinite number of solutions all of which fit the data equally well. We cannot determine which of these solutions best represents the parameters most likely to have generated the outcome data on the basis of model fit, and model fit is how such parameter estimates are typically determined in statistical analyses. It is this fit criterion that allows the researcher to point to a unique solution that provides an unbiased estimate of the underlying parameters (given the specification).

2.4 Generalized Linear Models

Although I have focused on the properties of the solutions to the APC multiple-classification model in the classic context of least squares solutions to the normal equations, this discussion can be extended to analyses based on generalized linear models. These models include Poisson regression that is often used to analyze APC multiple-classification models. The key to this extension is that generalized linear models treat the dependent variable as a linear function of the independent variables; that is, $g(E(Y_{ij})) = Xb$, where $(E(Y_{ij})$ is the expected value of the outcome variable for the ijth cell of the age–period table and g is the link function.[*]

In terms of identification in the generalized linear model approach, X has a rank deficiency of one and the identification problem is the same when

---

[*] For a comprehensive discussion of generalized linear models, see McCullagh and Nelder (1989).

generalized linear models or ordinary least squares (OLS) models are used. There is a single linear dependency in the matrix of independent variables so that we can write $Xv = \mathbf{0}$, with v being unique up to multiplication by a scalar (s): $Xsv = 0$. Because of this linear dependency, a best fitting solution to $g(E(Y_{ij})) = Xb_{c1}^0$ cannot be distinguished from the solution $g(E(Y_{ij})) = Xb_{c1}^0 + Xsv$ or in the notation that emphasizes the line of solutions $g(E(Y_{ij})) = X(b_{c1}^0 + sv)$. The generalized linear model solutions, in the rank deficient by one situation, lie on a line of solutions: $b_c^0 = b_{c1}^0 + sv$. There are an infinite number of solutions. These solutions lie on a line and differ from one another by the appropriate scalar times the null vector. Given the large number of observations on which the cell sizes for the age–period table are typically based, the results of using OLS regression with the logged cell rates as the dependent variable and the results of using Poisson regression are often quite similar (O'Brien 2000).

2.5 Null Vector

The null vector for a linearly coded APC model is easily derived by inspecting the columns of X. For example, from Table 2.1 for the deviation data we see that Age – Period + Cohort = zero, so we could use $(1, -1, 1)'$ for the null vector. If the X-matrix of independent variables in raw score form were used, a column of ones would be added before the age variable. Then the null vector for this X-matrix would be $(0, 1, -1, 1)'$. The dot product of each row of this X-matrix times this vector is zero and this means that $Xv = \mathbf{0}$. The null vector is unique up to multiplication by a scalar so this null vector could be represented as $(0, -1, 1, -1)'$ or by $(0, 3, -3, 3)'$. Typically, it is more difficult to determine the null vector in the case of a categorically coded matrix of independent variables. Kupper et al. (1980), however, provide a formula for determining the null vector for any age–period table for effect-coded independent variables (this formula is included in Appendix A2.2). Appendix A2.2 also includes a method for determining the null vector for the dummy-variable-coded independent variables.

A couple of examples of null vectors when using effect coding and a couple of examples when using dummy variable coding follow. The order of the elements is (intercept element, age elements, period elements, and cohort elements) where the reference categories are omitted, since they are not included as columns of X. The null vector, when effect coding is used for a 4 × 4 age–period table and the final element of each factor is used as a reference category, is $(0; -1.5, -0.5, .05; 1.5, 0.5, -0.5; -3, -2, -1, 0, 1, 2)'$. For conceptual convenience, I have used semicolons to separate the intercept element from the age elements, from the period elements, and from the cohort elements. The null vector for X with a 5 × 3 age–period table when using effect coding is (0; −2, −1, 0, 1; 1, 0; −3, −2, −1, 0, 1, 2)′. These null vector elements are derived using the general formula found in Kupper et al. (1983), which appears in Appendix A2.2 (Equation A2.2.1).

Note two characteristics of the null vector in the effect-coded situation. First, the null vector element for the intercept is always zero. To show the second characteristic, the concept of the "extended null vector" is helpful. In this conceptualization, the null vector is extended to include the reference categories in an intuitive manner. For example, in the 4×4 age–period table situation, the null vector includes an element for age4 that is coded as 1.5, an element for period4 coded as −1.5, and an element for cohort7 coded as 3. This results in an extended null vector of (0; −1.5, −0.5; .05, 1.5; 1.5, 0.5, −0.5, −1.5; −3, −2, −1, 0, 1, 2, 3)′.[*] Using the extended null vector, we note that there is a relationship between the age, period, and cohort null vector elements that represent a specific cell in the age–period table. The general rule is that for any of the age, period, and cohort elements of the null vector/extended null vector *intercept* + *age*$_i$ + *period*$_j$ + *cohort*$_{ij}$ = 0, where *cohort*$_{ij}$ stands for the cohort associated with the *ij*th cell of the age–period table.

Finding the null vector for dummy variable coding can be accomplished using two formulas for deriving the null vector elements that appears in Appendix A2.2 (Equations A2.2.2 and A2.2.3).[†] In the 4×4 age–period table situation, the null vector for dummy variable coding is (3; −3, −2, −1; 3, 2, 1; −6, −5, −4, −3, −2, −1)′ and the extended null vector is (3; −3, −2, −1, 0; 3, 2, 1, 0; −6, −5, −4, −3, −2, −1, 0)′. For the 5 by 3 age–period table the null vector for the dummy variable coding is (4; −4, −3, −2, −1; 2, 1; −6, −5, −4, −3, −2, −1)′ and for the extended null vector it is (4; −4, −3, −2, −1, 0; 2, 1, 0; −6, −5, −4, −3, −2, −1, 0)′. Note two characteristics of the null vector for dummy variable coding. The first is that the null vector element for the intercept is not always zero. Second, for dummy variable coding, the general rule is that for any of the age, period, and cohort elements of the null vector/extended null vector *intercept* + *age*$_i$ + *period*$_j$ + *cohort*$_{ij}$ = 0.

For both the effect-coded and dummy-variable-coded cases, the null vector is unique up to multiplication by a scalar. Although effect coding is primarily used throughout this book, there is the same sort of pattern to the null vector elements when dummy variable coding is utilized: linear increases from the youngest to the oldest age group, linear decreases from the earliest to the most recent period, and linear increases from the earliest to the most recent cohort. Again these are unique up to multiplication by a scalar. Since the scalar can be negative, we say that the trend of the null vector elements is the same for age groups and cohorts, and opposite for periods. The null vectors

---

[*] This vector would serve as a null vector for the effect coded variables in an X-matrix that included columns for the reference categories.

[†] Another way to obtain the null vector, whether the independent variables are effect coded or dummy variable coded, is to find the eigenvector of the appropriately coded X′X-matrix that is associated with the zero eigenvalue. This is the null vector, and it is unique up to multiplication by a scalar.

for the effect- and dummy-coded variables have the same type of implica-tions for the relationships among solutions, $b_c^0 = b_{c1}^0 + sv$, where v is the null vector of effect-coded or dummy-coded age, period, and cohort variables.

2.6 Model Fit

The fit of the model to the observed data is the same for all of the con-strained estimators. That is, they each produce the same predicted val-ues. Perhaps the most general way to see this result relies on the fact that the solutions all lie on a line of solutions $b_c^0 = b_{c1}^0 + sv$. Since b_{c1}^0 produces a best fitting solution, the predicted values for the cells can be represented as $\hat{y} = X b_{c1}^0$. However, b_c^0 also produces a best fitting solution, since $Xsv = \mathbf{0}$, then $X b_c^0 = X b_{c1}^0 + Xsv = X b_{c1}^0 = \hat{y}$. This is the same for generalized linear mod-els where $g(E(Y_{ij})) = X b_c^0 = X b_{c1}^0 + Xsv = X b_{c1}^0 = \hat{y})$, since the expected value of the dependent variable is a linear function of the independent variables as described earlier. The predicted values of y will usually be different for the OLS and generalized linear model estimates (except when the general-ized linear model uses the identity link function and normal distribution function). For example, the solutions for the Poisson regression estimates will produce the same predicted values of y no matter which constraint is used, and the solutions for the OLS estimates produce, in general, a different set of predicted values for y that are the same no matter which constraint is used. This property of the equality of model fit for coefficient estimates based on different constraints is well known to APC analysts. It means that model fit cannot be used to choose between constrained regression estima-tors in such models.[*]

2.7 Solution Is Orthogonal to the Constraint

To set the constraint in the 4×4 age–period table situation that age1 = age2, the constraint would be $(0, 1, -1, 0, 0, \cdots, 0)'$. This is how the constraint is set in the Mazumdar, Li, and Bryce (1980) procedure or in a constrained regression program. The solution vector produced is $(b_0, b_1, b_2, b_3, \cdots, b_{12})'$ with $b_1 = b_2$. Because $b_1 = b_2$; the dot product $(0, 1, -1, 0, 0, \cdots, 0) \cdot (b_0, b_1, b_2, b_3, \cdots, b_{12})' = 0$. This generalizes, the constraint vector imposes the following requirement on the solution vector: the dot product of the constraint vector with the solution

---

[*] Throughout this chapter we consider only single constraints that just identify the APC model.

vector equals zero. Remembering that two vectors are orthogonal if their dot product is zero, we can write $c'b_c^0 = 0$.

2.8 Examining the Relationship between Solutions

For concreteness, an empirical example is used to illustrate several of the points related to the characteristics of constrained solutions in APC models. The data used are drawn from an article by Clayton and Schifflers (1987) that records the mortality rates (per 100,000) and the number of cases of breast cancer mortality in Japan during the period 1955–1979. The data are reproduced in Table 2.3. Clayton and Schifflers obtained the data from the World Health Organization mortality database. The data are presented in terms of an age–period table with 5-year age groupings (25–29, 30–34, ..., 75–79). The mortality data for these age groups are aggregated over 5-year periods (1955–1959, 1960–1964, ..., 1975–1979), and the rates are per 100,000 years of observation. These rates are approximately the yearly rate during these 5-year periods per 100,000 persons at risk in these age groups. The aggregation of the data across the 5-year periods leaves the years spanned by the birth cohort quite imprecise. For example, a person in the 25–29 age category in the period 1960–1964, could be born as early as 1930 and as late as 1939. Clayton and Schifflers label this cohort the 1930 cohort. This does not change the mechanics of the analysis. The "cell" corresponding to the earliest cohort

TABLE 2.3

Age-Specific Mortality Rates from Breast Cancer in Japan (per 100,000 Person Years of Observation) with the Number of Deaths in Parentheses

Age	Period									
	1955–1959		1960–1964		1965–1969		1970–1974		1975–1979	
25–29	0.44	(88)	0.38	(78)	0.46	(101)	0.55	(127)	0.68	(179)
30–34	1.69	(299)	1.69	(330)	1.75	(363)	2.31	(509)	2.52	(588)
35–39	4.01	(596)	3.90	(680)	4.11	(798)	4.44	(923)	4.80	(1056)
40–44	6.59	(874)	6.57	(962)	6.81	(1171)	7.79	(1497)	8.27	(1716)
45–49	8.51	(1022)	9.61	(1247)	9.96	(1429)	11.68	(1987)	12.51	(2398)
50–54	10.49	(1035)	10.8	(1258)	12.36	(1560)	14.59	(2079)	16.56	(2794)
55–59	11.36	(970)	11.51	(1087)	12.98	(1446)	14.97	(1828)	17.79	(2465)
60–64	12.03	(820)	10.67	(861)	12.67	(1126)	14.46	(1549)	16.42	(1962)
65–69	12.55	(678)	12.03	(738)	12.1	(878)	13.81	(1140)	16.46	(1683)
70–74	15.81	(640)	13.87	(628)	12.65	(656)	14.00	(900)	15.60	(1162)
75–79	17.97	(497)	15.62	(463)	15.83	(536)	15.71	(644)	16.52	(865)

Source: Data from Clayton, D., and E. Schifflers, 1987, Models for temporal variation in cancer rates II: Age-period-cohort models, *Statistics in Medicine* 6:468–81, Table 1.

is the lower left-hand cell; it corresponds to the cell for the oldest age group (75–79) and earliest period (1955–1959). Given how the age groups, periods, and cohorts are designated in this example, the linear dependency between age, period, and cohort exists no matter what the labels for the cell or cohorts. The corresponding cohorts are on the diagonals of the table (upper left-hand to lower right-hand side).[*]

We begin by analyzing these data using Poisson regression. Clayton and Schifflers (1987) used this form of analysis when working with these data. For Poisson regression we need to know the number of people who died in each of these categories. That data is provided in Table 2.3 in parentheses; for example, 88 such deaths occurred for those age 25–29 during the 5 years from 1955 through 1959. We also need to know the number of person–years of exposure or observation. For these data we can calculate the number of years of exposure as the number of deaths in each age–period-specific category times 100,000 divided by the rate per 100,000. For those 25–29 in 1955–1959 the number of person years of observation is 20,000,000 [(= 88 × 100,000)/.44]. This number represents the person–years of risk in a cell and is used as the "exposure" in the Poisson regression. Poisson regression analysis will be used throughout this chapter and the book as an illustration of generalized linear models and their properties in terms of constrained regression, estimable functions, variance decomposition, and so forth. For simplicity, I forego testing whether to use negative binomial regression or whether some other form of analysis meets the assumptions better and then switching between these forms of analysis. OLS analysis will also be used and compared and contrasted with Poisson regression results.

The results from the Poisson regression analysis of the breast cancer mortality data appear in Table 2.4. The second through fifth columns of the table show the results from the Poisson regression analysis using four different constraints: constraining the first two age categories to be equal, constraining the second and third periods to be equal, constraining the effects of the sixth and seventh cohorts to be equal, and constraining the solution to be orthogonal to the null vector (the intrinsic estimator [IE]/Moore–Penrose solution). The final column is the extended null vector for the design matrix for this 11 × 5 age–period matrix that has been effect coded. The "extended elements," which are not part of the null vector, are in italics.

The first thing to note is that the solutions can differ dramatically depending upon the constraint used. For instance, the age 25–29 and age 30–34 effects are strongly positive for the age1 = age2 constrained solution and negative for all of the other solutions. Other constraints would show different patterns. True to their name, "constrained solutions" work in terms of implementing their constraints. We see this in the first three columns of solutions where the age 25–29 and age 30–34 effects are equal for the age constraint;

---

[*] Later I will show how combining cohorts while leaving the coding of the age groups and periods the same can identify the model, but this change imposes a constraint on the model.

TABLE 2.4

Poisson Regression Analysis of the Japanese Breast Cancer Mortality Data in Table 2.3 (Effect Coded)

	age1 = age2	per2 = per3	coh6 = coh7	Intrinsic Estimator	Extended Null Vector[a]
Intercept	−9.5250	−9.5250	−9.5250	−9.5250	0
age 25–29	4.3869	−3.0527	−2.5052	−2.3251	−5
age 30–34	4.3869	−1.5648	−1.1268	−0.9827	−4
age 35–39	3.7316	−0.7322	−0.4037	−0.2956	−3
age 40–44	2.8401	−0.1357	0.0833	0.1553	−2
age 45–49	1.7932	0.3053	0.4148	0.4508	−1
age 50–54	0.6071	0.6071	0.6071	0.6071	0
age 55–59	−0.7279	0.7600	0.6505	0.6145	1
age 60–64	−2.1619	0.8140	0.5950	0.5229	2
age 65–69	−3.5689	0.8949	0.5664	0.4583	3
age 70–74	−4.9645	0.9871	0.5491	0.4050	4
age 75–79	−6.3226	1.1170	0.5695	0.3894	5
period 1955–59	−2.9489	0.0270	−0.1920	−0.2641	2
period 1960–64	−1.5336	−0.0457	−0.1552	−0.1912	1
period 1965–69	−0.0457	−0.0457	−0.0457	−0.0457	0
period 1970–74	1.5033	0.0153	0.1248	0.1609	−1
period 1975–79	3.0249	0.0491	0.2681	0.3401	−2
cohort 1875	10.1722	−0.2433	0.5232	0.7754	−7
cohort 1880	8.6564	−0.2711	0.3859	0.6020	−6
cohort 1885	7.1102	−0.3294	0.2181	0.3982	−5
cohort 1890	5.5908	−0.3609	0.0771	0.2212	−4
cohort 1895	4.1083	−0.3555	−0.0270	0.0811	−3
cohort 1900	2.7162	−0.2597	−0.0407	0.0314	−2
cohort 1905	1.3378	−0.1502	−0.0407	−0.0046	−1
cohort 1910	−0.0322	−0.0322	−0.0322	−0.0322	0
cohort 1915	−1.4142	0.0737	−0.0358	−0.0718	1
cohort 1920	−2.8307	0.1451	−0.0739	−0.1459	2
cohort 1925	−4.2782	0.1856	−0.1429	−0.2510	3
cohort 1930	−5.7432	0.2085	−0.2295	−0.3736	4
cohort 1935	−7.1322	0.3074	−0.2401	−0.4202	5
cohort 1940	−8.4756	0.4519	−0.2051	−0.4212	6
cohort 1945	−9.7854	0.6300	−0.1365	−0.3887	7

[a] The "extended" elements in the null vector are italicized.

the 1960–1964 and 1965–1969 period effects are equal for the period constraint; and the 1900 and 1905 cohort effects are equal for the cohort constraint. These equalities are implicit in these constraints. For example, since the constraint for age1 = age2 is (0, 1, − 1, 0, 0, ..., 0) and this vector times the solution vector for this constraint must equal zero, this requires that the age1 coefficient equal the age2 coefficient. The pattern of the IE solution is also implied by its constraint. The constraint vector is the null vector and the dot product of the IE solution vector times the null vector equals zero. This is another way of saying that each of these solutions is orthogonal to its constraint. If the dot product between two vectors is zero, then the two vectors are orthogonal. Orthogonality is described in greater detail in the next chapter, which focuses on the geometry of the APC model.

To show that these solutions lie on a line, it is necessary to show that they differ from one another by sv and that is the case with the four constrained solutions to the Poisson regression in Table 2.4. To move from the age1 = age2 solution to the period2 = period3 solution, we add 1.4879 times the null vector elements (or extended null vector elements if we want the solutions for the reference categories) to elements of the age1 = age2 constrained solution: $b_{p2=p3} = b_{a1=a2} + 1.4879 \cdot v$. To move from the age1 = age2 constrained solution to the coh6 = coh7 solution $s = 1.3784$, and to move from the age1 = age2 solution to the IE solution $s = 1.3424$. These solutions lie on a line in multidimensional (29 dimensional) solution space.[*] We also note that the solutions for the intercepts is the same across all of the constrained solutions, as are the solutions for age 50–54, period 65–69, and cohort 1910. This occurs because the null vector elements corresponding to each of these is zero and the constrained solutions differ from each other by sv.

Each of these solutions fits the data equally well. For each of these constrained solutions the log likelihood is −249.482. The deviance goodness of fit is 30.46 with 27 degrees of freedom and Pearson's goodness of fit is 30.53 with 27 degrees of freedom, indicating that the model fits the data very well. The probability associated with each of these goodness of fit measures is greater than .29. The predicted values for the number of cases in each cell of the age–period table are the same regardless of the constraint used. Even though each of these solutions fits the data equally well, the solutions diverge in terms of their estimated effect parameters. The researcher will need to bring some other insight (substantive knowledge/theory) into this mix if she is to choose among these solutions or some other constrained solutions as approximating the parameters that generated the outcome values.

Table 2.5 presents the results of using an OLS regression with the data in Table 2.3, but the dependent variable is the log of the rate of breast cancer. This is another common form for the analysis of such data and it is typical that the results are similar to those from Poisson regression (O'Brien 2000).[†] This similarity holds in this case with only the intercepts showing a major

---

[*] Twenty-nine because there are 29 elements in b_c^0, the solution vector, which matches the 29 columns of X. Table 2.4 reports 32 coefficients, which include the reference categories, whose values are derived from the age, period, and cohort elements in the solution vector.

[†] It is important to log the dependent variable in the OLS regression. These rates based on counts are typically positively skewed. Logging the rates establishes the same "link function" that is used with Poisson regression. The similarity of the Poisson and OLS regression results is helped by large counts in each cell.

TABLE 2.5

OLS Regression Analysis of the Japanese Logged Breast Cancer Mortality Rates per 100,000 in Table 2.3 (Effect Coded)

	age1 = age2	per2 = per3	coh6 = coh7	Intrinsic Estimator	Extended Null Vector[a]
Intercept	1.9887	1.9887	1.9887	1.9887	0
age 25–29	4.3715	–3.1031	–2.5256	–2.3302	–5
age 30–34	4.3715	–1.6082	–1.1462	–0.9899	–4
age 35–39	3.7325	–0.7522	–0.4057	–0.2885	–3
age 40–44	2.8443	–0.1455	0.0855	0.1636	–2
age 45–49	1.7936	0.2987	0.4142	0.4533	–1
age 50–54	0.6057	0.6057	0.6057	0.6057	0
age 55–59	–0.7256	0.7693	0.6538	0.6147	1
age 60–64	–2.1559	0.8340	0.6029	0.5248	2
age 65–69	–3.5681	0.9166	0.5701	0.4529	3
age 70–74	–4.9544	1.0253	0.5632	0.4070	4
age 75–79	–6.3151	1.1594	0.5819	0.3866	5
period 1955–59	–2.9443	0.0456	–0.1855	–0.2636	2
period 1960–64	–1.5381	–0.0432	–0.1587	–0.1977	1
period 1965–69	–0.0432	–0.0432	–0.0432	–0.0432	0
period 1970–74	1.5077	0.0128	0.1283	0.1674	–1
period 1975–79	3.0178	0.0279	0.2590	0.3371	–2
cohort 1875	10.1594	–0.3050	0.5035	0.7770	–7
cohort 1880	8.6418	–0.3277	0.3654	0.5997	–6
cohort 1885	7.1061	–0.3685	0.2091	0.4044	–5
cohort 1890	5.5808	–0.3989	0.0632	0.2194	–4
cohort 1895	4.1020	–0.3828	–0.0362	0.0809	–3
cohort 1900	2.7120	–0.2778	–0.0468	0.0314	–2
cohort 1905	1.3326	–0.1623	–0.0468	–0.0077	–1
cohort 1910	–0.0277	–0.0277	–0.0277	–0.0277	0
cohort 1915	–1.4131	0.0819	–0.0337	–0.0727	1
cohort 1920	–2.8445	0.1454	–0.0856	–0.1638	2
cohort 1925	–4.2721	0.2127	–0.1339	–0.2511	3
cohort 1930	–5.7559	0.2238	–0.2383	–0.3945	4
cohort 1935	–7.0982	0.3764	–0.2012	–0.3965	5
cohort 1940	–8.4597	0.5098	–0.1833	–0.4177	6
cohort 1945	–9.7636	0.7008	–0.1078	–0.3812	7

[a] The "extended" elements in the null vector are italicized.

difference. These OLS solutions all lie on the same line of solutions (a different line than the Poisson regression solutions). Here to move from the age1 = age2 constrained solution to the period2 = period3 constrained solution, $s = 1.4949$; from age1 = age2 to the cohort6 = cohort7 solution, $s = 1.3794$; and from the age1 = age2 constrained solution to the IE solution, $s = 1.3403$.

Again no matter what the constraint, the solutions for the intercept, age 50–54, period 65–69, and cohort 1910 are the same, since the null vector elements associated with these coefficients are zeros. Each of the solutions is orthogonal to its constraint. The fit of these constrained models is the same. They predict the same age–period rates for the cells, the model and residual sums of squares are identical, and $R^2 = .9994$ for each of the models. This excellent fit of the predicted to observed values of the dependent variable in APC models was commented on by Kupper et al. (1983): "the squared multiple correlation coefficient R^2 is fairly close to 1, a result which seems to occur not infrequently in practice" (p. 2797).

For comparison the results for the same two analyses using dummy variable coding are reported in Tables 2.6 and 2.7. Although effect coding is typically used in this book, dummy variable coding appears at times in the literature and the comparison is enlightening. The fit of the Poisson analyses for the effect-coded variables and the dummy-variable-coded variables is the same; the predicted number of deaths in each cell of the age–period table is the same not only across all of the constrained estimates, but whether dummy coding or effect coding is used. The same is the case when we compare the OLS regression results with one another. The fit does not depend upon the coding or the constraint used. The values of s for moving from the age1 = age2 solution to each of the other solutions is the same for effect coding and dummy variable coding in the Poisson analyses results. This result holds for the OLS regressions; the values of s for moving from the age1 = age2 solution to each of the other solutions are the same for effect coding and dummy variable coding. With the exception of the results associated with the IE these results are reassuring. In terms of substantive conclusions, the results from the Poisson regression and from OLS regression do not depend upon using effect coding or dummy variable coding.[*]

For the classic constrained estimators, the effect-coded results can be transformed to the dummy-variable-coded results by simply adding or subtracting coefficients. The transformation from the effect-coded coefficients to dummy-variable-coded coefficients can be accomplished by (1) adding the intercept coefficient and the effect coefficient values associated with the reference categories to produce the intercept for the dummy-coded solution,

---

[*] I calculated the IE with the dummy variable coding by rotating the age1=age2 solution based on dummy variable coding so that it was orthogonal to the null vector. This technique, the "s-constraint" approach, is discussed in Chapter 7.

TABLE 2.6

Poisson Regression Analysis of the Japanese Breast Cancer Mortality Data in Table 2.3 (Dummy Variable Coded)

	age1 = age2	per2 = per3	coh6 = coh7	Intrinsic Estimator	Extended Null Vector[a]
Intercept	−22.6081	−7.7289	−8.8239	−8.3205	10
age 25–29	10.7095	−4.1697	−3.0747	−3.5781	−10
age 30–34	10.7095	−2.6818	−1.6963	−2.1493	−9
age 35–39	10.0541	−1.8492	−0.9732	−1.3759	−8
age 40–44	9.1627	−1.2527	−0.4863	−0.8386	−7
age 45–49	8.1158	−0.8117	−0.1547	−0.4567	−6
age 50–54	6.9296	−0.5100	0.0375	−0.2142	−5
age 55–59	5.5947	−0.3570	0.0810	−0.1203	−4
age 60–64	4.1607	−0.3031	0.0254	−0.1256	−3
age 65–69	2.7537	−0.2222	−0.0032	−0.1039	−2
age 70–74	1.3580	−0.1299	−0.0204	−0.0707	−1
age 75–79	0.0000	0.0000	0.0000	0.0000	0
period 1955–59	−5.9738	−0.0221	−0.4601	−0.2588	4
period 1960–64	−4.5585	−0.0947	−0.4232	−0.2722	3
period 1965–69	−3.0706	−0.0947	−0.3137	−0.2130	2
period 1970–74	−1.5216	−0.0337	−0.1432	−0.0929	1
period 1975–79	0.0000	0.0000	1.3403	0.6356	0
cohort 1875	19.9576	−0.8732	0.6597	0.0000	−14
cohort 1880	18.4418	−0.9011	0.5224	0.0053	−13
cohort 1885	16.8957	−0.9594	0.3546	−0.0816	−12
cohort 1890	15.3763	−0.9909	0.2136	−0.1991	−11
cohort 1895	13.8937	−0.9855	0.1095	−0.2898	−10
cohort 1900	12.5016	−0.8897	0.0958	−0.3435	−9
cohort 1905	11.1232	−0.7802	0.0000	−0.3069	−8
cohort 1910	9.7532	−0.6622	0.1043	−0.2480	−7
cohort 1915	8.3712	−0.5563	0.1007	−0.2013	−6
cohort 1920	6.9547	−0.4849	0.0626	−0.1891	−5
cohort 1925	5.5073	−0.4444	−0.0064	−0.2077	−4
cohort 1930	4.0423	−0.4215	−0.0930	−0.2440	−3
cohort 1935	2.6532	−0.3226	−0.1036	−0.2043	−2
cohort 1940	1.3098	−0.1781	−0.0686	−0.1189	−1
cohort 1945	0.0000	0.0000	0.0000	0.0000	0

[a] The "extended" elements in the null vector are italicizedTable 2.7 OLS regression analysis of the Japanese logged breast cancer mortality rates per 100,000 in Table 2.3 (dummy variable coded).

TABLE 2.7

OLS Regression Analysis of the Japanese Logged Breast Cancer Mortality Rates per 100,000 in Table 2.3 (Dummy-Variable Coded)

	age1 = age2	per2 = per3	coh6 = coh7	Intrinsic Estimator	Extended Null Vector[a]
Intercept	−11.0723	3.8769	2.7218	2.3327	10
age 25–29	10.6866	−4.2625	−3.1075	−2.7184	−10
age 30–34	10.6866	−2.7676	−1.7281	−1.3779	−9
age 35–39	10.0477	−1.9117	−0.9876	−0.6763	−8
age 40–44	9.1594	−1.3050	−0.4964	−0.2240	−7
age 45–49	8.1087	−0.8607	−0.1677	0.0658	−6
age 50–54	6.9209	−0.5537	0.0238	0.2184	−5
age 55–59	5.5895	−0.3902	0.0719	0.2275	−4
age 60–64	4.1593	−0.3255	0.0210	0.1377	−3
age 65–69	2.7470	−0.2428	−0.0118	0.0660	−2
age 70–74	1.3607	−0.1342	−0.0187	0.0202	−1
age 75–79	0.0000	0.0000	0.0000	0.0000	0
period 1955–59	−5.9620	0.0176	−0.4444	−0.6000	4
period 1960–64	−4.5558	−0.0711	−0.4176	−0.5343	3
period 1965–69	−3.0609	−0.0711	−0.3021	−0.3799	2
period 1970–74	−1.5100	−0.0151	−0.1306	−0.1695	1
period 1975–79	0.0000	0.0000	0.0000	1.1560	0
cohort 1875	19.9230	−1.0058	0.6113	0.0000	−14
cohort 1880	18.4054	−1.0285	0.4732	0.9790	−13
cohort 1885	16.8697	−1.0692	0.3169	0.7838	−12
cohort 1890	15.3444	−1.0997	0.1709	0.5989	−11
cohort 1895	13.8656	−1.0835	0.0715	0.4606	−10
cohort 1900	12.4757	−0.9786	0.0610	0.4112	−9
cohort 1905	11.0963	−0.8631	0.0610	0.3723	−8
cohort 1910	9.7360	−0.7285	0.0801	0.3525	−7
cohort 1915	8.3506	−0.6189	0.0741	0.3076	−6
cohort 1920	6.9192	−0.5554	0.0221	0.2167	−5
cohort 1925	5.4915	−0.4881	−0.0261	0.1295	−4
cohort 1930	4.0077	−0.4770	−0.1305	−0.0138	−3
cohort 1935	2.6654	−0.3244	−0.0934	−0.0156	−2
cohort 1940	1.3039	−0.1910	−0.0755	−0.0366	−1
cohort 1945	0.0000	0.0000	0.0000	0.0000	0

[a] The "extended" elements in the null vector are italicized.

then (2) subtracting the age reference category solution for the effect-coded data from each of the effect-coded age solutions; subtracting the period reference category solution from each of the period solutions; and subtracting the cohort reference category solution from each of the cohort solutions to produce the dummy-coded age, period, cohort solutions. It is a simple matter to transform the dummy-variable solutions to the effect-coded solutions.

One last comment on both the dummy-variable and the effect-coded solutions. For the dummy-variable solution the coefficients associated with age, period, and cohort categories are relative to the reference category. A coefficient for age 30–34 of 10.6866 for the age1 = age2 solution in Table 2.7 is relative to the reference category of age 75–79. If the reference category were age 35–39, the effect associated with the dummy coded age 30–34 variable would be 0.6389 (the difference between the age 30–34 coefficient minus the age 35–39 coefficient). One cannot simply associate the size of the effect with the size of the dummy variable coefficient. The significance tests associated with the dummy variables are based on the difference between the categorical variable and the reference category. With effect coding the intercept is the grand mean. The age, period, and cohort coefficients represent the difference from the grand mean of being in that category (controlling for the other independent variables in the model). The significance tests associated with the categorical variables test whether the coefficient is significantly different from the grand mean but not from the other categorical variables. A different test is needed to make that comparison.

If a model provided unbiased or nearly unbiased estimates of the parameters that generated the y values, a focus on the differences between these coefficients would make sense. Without these estimates, comparisons of the differences between coefficients make little sense, as can be seen from the results using different constraints. These comparisons depend upon the constraint used. It is for this reason (in part) that I do not report the significance levels for the categorical coefficients in this chapter.

2.9 Differences between Constrained Solutions as Rotations of Solutions

The constrained solutions differ from one another by sv; with s being a scalar. The elements of the null vector, as we have seen, are linear within age groups, periods, and cohorts and on an equal interval scale. The sign of the trend represented by the null vector elements is the same for age groups and cohorts and of the opposite sign for the periods. A solution using a new constraint will move the trend in the coefficients for age and cohort in the same direction and the trend for the coefficients for periods in the opposite direction. More concretely for the breast cancer data from Clayton and Schifflers (1987) using effect coding, the extended null vector is (0; −5, −4, −3, −2, −1, 0, 1, 2, 3, 4, 5; 2, 1, 0, −1, −2; −7, −6, −5, −4, −3, −2, −1, 0, 1, 2, 3, 4, 5, 6, 7)'. It exhibits this linear equal interval coding for ages, periods, and cohorts. The vector of solutions changes from one solution to another by adding s times this vector

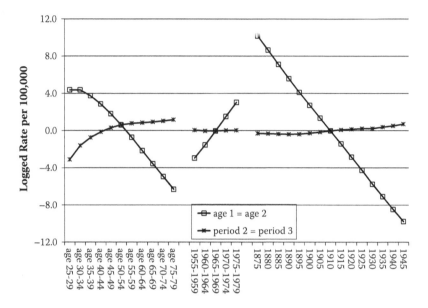

FIGURE 2.1
Effect-coded coefficients for mortality due to breast cancer under two different constraints analyzing the logged rates.

to a solution. That addition changes the trends in age, period, and cohort coefficients in a systematic manner (illustrated in Figure 2.1).

Figure 2.1 demonstrates this shift in trends using the data for the age1 = age2 constraint and for the period2 = period3 constraint from Table 2.5 for the effect-coded OLS analysis of the logged rates of breast cancer mortality. Given our coding of the null vector,[*] if s is positive for moving from the solutions for the age constraint to the period constraint, the slope of the age coefficients will increase when using the period constraint. The same is the case for the cohort coefficients and the opposite is the case for the period coefficients. Figure 2.1 clearly shows this shift. The curves are the same except that they have different linear trends. The first age coefficient based on the period constraint is 7.4746 less than the first age coefficient based on the age constraint, which is $s = 1.4949$ times the null vector element for age1 (−5). This shift occurs because the age constraint in this case makes the coefficients for the first two age groups the same. That fixes the trends for all ages and for the period and cohort effects. The second set of solutions is constrained so that coefficients for period2 and period3 are equal (as can be seen from their equality in

---

[*] Note there is some degree of arbitrariness in our coding of the null vector (resulting from its uniqueness up to multiplication by a scalar). If we divide the null vector (as we have coded it) by 2, it is still the null vector. We would have to multiply s by 2 to have the same effect in moving from one solution to another. If we divided our representation of the null vector by −2, it would still be the null vector, but we would need to multiply s by −2 to have the same effect in moving from one solution to another. Such changes would have no effect on Figure 2.1.

Figure 2.1). This sets the trend for periods and, thus, for ages and for cohorts. This shift in the linear trends of age, period, and cohort coefficients determines the difference between the solutions and leads some researchers to say that it is the linear trends that are not identified in the APC model.

2.10 Solutions Ignoring One or More of the Age, Period, or Cohort Factors

A common strategy used when analyzing an age–period table is to ignore the cohort variable and proceed with an analysis that includes only the age and period categorical variables. This strategy ignores the potential impact of cohorts on the relationship between age groups and periods. Most importantly, it assumes that any linear trend in cohort effects is zero. A different strategy that results in the same potential problem is the recommendation to test to see if a two-factor model (Age–Period or Age–Cohort or Period–Cohort) fits the data nearly as well as the APC model. If it does, the recommendation is to use that two-factor model (Yang and Land 2013a, 2013b). The results of such an analysis appear in the first column of results in Table 2.8, and I have included the implied cohort effects of zero in italics. The age–period model institutes a series of *implicit constraints* with many more constraints than the constrained models that we have been using. It constrains cohort1 = 0, cohort2 = 0, …, cohort14 = 0 by simply not including these categorical variables in the model. It does not fit the data as well as the constrained models that we have been using, which use only a single constraint to identify the model.

The second column of results in Table 2.8 contains a solution based on a just-identifying constraint of the type we have been using. It constrains the slope of the cohort effect coefficients to be zero.* This is one of the constrained solutions on the line of solutions; note that it shares the same intercept as those solutions as well as the age 50–54, period 1965–1969, and 1910 cohort coefficients (Table 2.5). We can find values of s that will transform any solution to the line of solutions to this solution. This solution is related to Figure 2.1, since it is the solution we would obtain if we "rotated" linear components of the cohorts in Figure 2.1 to have no slope for the cohort coefficients.

Even though both of the models in Table 2.8 constrain the slope of cohort effects to be zero, the solutions differ between the Age–Period model and the APC model with the zero linear trend in cohorts constraint. Examining the column that contains the solution for the zero linear trend in cohorts constraint, we see that this does not eliminate the cohort effects. These nonlinear

---

* The constraint is based on a vector of all zeros except for the cohort elements that are coded −14, −13, …, −1, that is, c = (0, 0, …0, −14, −13, …, −1)′.

TABLE 2.8

Comparison of the Age–Period Model and the Zero
Linear Trend for Cohorts Constrained Model

Effect Coefficients	Age–Period Model	Zero Linear Trend for Cohorts Constraint
Intercept	1.9529	1.9887
age 25–29	–2.6626	–2.7253
age 30–34	–1.2788	–1.3059
age 35–39	–0.5084	–0.5256
age 40–44	0.0175	0.0056
age 45–49	0.3845	0.3743
age 50–54	0.5935	0.6057
age 55–59	0.6514	0.6937
age 60–64	0.6199	0.6828
age 65–69	0.6344	0.6900
age 70–74	0.7100	0.7230
age 75–79	0.8387	0.7817
1955–1959	–0.0832	–0.1056
1960–1964	–0.1239	–0.1187
1965–1969	–0.0599	–0.0432
1970–1974	0.0759	0.0884
1975–1979	0.1910	0.1791
1875	*0.0000*	0.2239
1880	*0.0000*	0.1257
1885	*0.0000*	0.0093
1890	*0.0000*	–0.0966
1895	*0.0000*	–0.1561
1900	*0.0000*	–0.1267
1905	*0.0000*	–0.0867
1910	*0.0000*	–0.0277
1915	*0.0000*	0.0063
1920	*0.0000*	–0.0057
1925	*0.0000*	–0.0140
1930	*0.0000*	–0.0785
1935	*0.0000*	–0.0014
1940	*0.0000*	0.0564
1945	*0.0000*	0.1719

cohort effects have a distinct pattern with a drop from the 1875 cohort to the 1895 cohort, a rise in cohort effects until the 1915 cohort, followed by a decrease to the 1930 cohort, and an increase through the 1945 cohort. The age and period effects are controlled for these fluctuations of cohort effects in the zero linear trend for cohorts model, while there is no control for these nonlinear cohort effects in the Age–Period model. The most important point is that leaving cohorts out of Age–Period analysis and thus ignoring the confounding effects of cohorts is not a solution to the APC problem. It assumes that there are no linear effects of cohorts: no cohort effects at all on the outcome variable. This problem exists in not only the two-factor age–period model, but also in the two factor age-cohort and period-cohort models. In each of these cases an assumption is made regarding the effects of cohorts or periods or ages. As I will discuss at length in later chapters the two-factor models absorb any linear effect of the third factor. We cannot judge the importance of the linear trend in the third factor by comparing the two-factor model to the three-factor (APC) model since the two-factor model takes credit for any linear trend in the third factor due to the data generating parameters. The zeros in the result column for the Age-Period model are italicized because they are implied by not including the cohort category variables in the model.

One-factor models have analogous problems. When examining the age distribution of breast cancer mortality in a cross-sectional study, period is controlled for by holding it constant. This may seem to be a solution to our problem, but each of the age groups is represented by a different birth cohort. When examining the age distribution in a specific period, care must be taken not to attribute that distribution to the effects of age alone. In this cross-sectional case, the effects of age are completely confounded with the effects of cohorts. Each age group represents a different cohort.

To investigate the potential impact of this confounding, the age effects for the 1960–1964 period are examined. The cross-sectional age effects were obtained by regressing the logged age-specific rates for the breast cancer reported in Table 2.3 for the period 1960–64 on the effect-coded age categories. These "age effects" appear in the second column in Table 2.9 and do not control for the potential impact of cohort effects. The potential impacts of cohort effects on these cross-sectional age effects are shown using two different constraints on the APC models: cohort6 = cohort7 and period2 = period3. To make these age-effects more comparable to the age effects for the 1960–64 period, the 1960–64 period effects from each of the APC constrained models were added to the age effects in these models. Note that the age effects are controlled for cohort effects (as estimated under the constrained solution) in each of these constrained models.

For each of the constraints and for the cross-sectional data the age effects increase from age 25–29 through age 55–59. Then for the estimates based on the cohort6 = cohort7 constraint, the age effect decreases slightly and remains fairly level. This contrasts with the estimates based on the period2 = period3 constraint. In this case, the age effects increase monotonically from age 25–29 through 75–79. For the cross-sectional data, there is a drop from age 55–59 to age 60–64 and then the age effects continue their upward trend through age 75–79. Each of these estimates makes different assumptions about the cohort effects. The cross-sectional analysis assumes that the cohort effects are zero. The constrained estimates assume the cohort effects coincide with what they

TABLE 2.9

Cross-Sectional Analysis of the 1900–84 Breast Cancer Mortality Data: Estimated Age Effects Using Cross-Sectional Data Compared with the Age Effects Using Different Constraints in an APC Model

	Age Effects 1960–64	Age–Period–Cohort-Based Age Effects	
		Cohort6 = Cohort7	Period2 = Period3
age 25–29	−2.797	−2.684	−3.146
age 30–34	−1.304	−1.305	−1.651
age 35–39	−0.468	−0.564	−0.795
age 40–44	0.053	−0.073	−0.189
age 45–49	0.434	0.256	0.256
age 50–54	0.551	0.447	0.563
age 55–59	0.614	0.495	0.726
age 60–64	0.538	0.444	0.791
age 65–69	0.658	0.411	0.873
age 70–74	0.801	0.405	0.982
age 75–79	0.920	0.423	1.116

Source: Data from Clayton, D., and E. Schifflers, 1987, Models for temporal variation in cancer rates II: Age-period-cohort models, *Statistics in Medicine* 6:468–81, Table 1.

are estimated to be under the particular constraint. All three estimates of the age effects make an assumption about the cohort effects.

Figure 2.2 shows the age distributions of breast cancer in 1960–64 based on the cross-sectional data and the age distribution after "corrections for cohort effects." Our procedure was to add the intercept to the age-effect coefficients for the cross-sectional analysis and to exponentiate these sums to "estimate" age distribution. Given this cross-sectional data, this simply corresponds to the age distribution of breast cancer for 1960–64 in Table 2.3. To obtain the two age distributions controlling for cohort effects (as estimated by those models), the intercept in the model and the period effect for 1960–64 were added to each of the age effects. These sums were then exponentiated to obtain the age distribution for the 1960–64 period controlling for cohort effects (as estimated under each of these two constraints). Not surprisingly, this pattern in the age distributions is similar to that for the age effects in Table 2.9. Figure 2.2 shows how cohort effects can shape cross-sectional age distributions in a dramatic manner.

This odyssey into the relationships among solutions using empirical data was designed to provide concrete illustrations of many of the characteristics of APC models discussed at the beginning of this chapter. There are a few more topics to be addressed before moving to the geometry of APC models (Chapter 3). These are related to some of the topics discussed earlier. This chapter concludes with an empirical example of a plausible constraint.

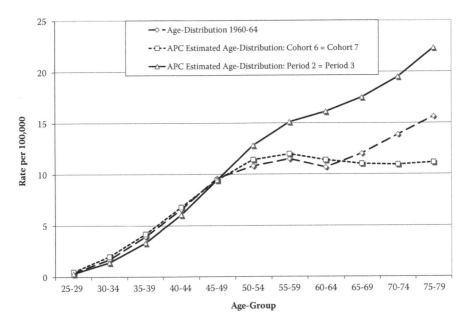

FIGURE 2.2
Age effects on breast cancer mortality rates in Japan 1960–1964 based on cross-sectional data and the age effects for 1960–1964 controlling for cohort effects.

2.11 Bias: Constrained Estimates and the Data Generating Parameters

A substantive researcher wants to know how the outcome variable was generated. What are the values of the age, period, and cohort parameters that generated the outcome variable (e.g., the mortality rate, attitudes toward same-sex marriage, or the unemployment rate)? Did the cohort effect peak with the earliest cohort or the sixth earliest cohort? Is there a positive trend in the effects of periods over the time covered by the study? What is the relationship between the outcome variable and the age, period, and cohort categories associated with how the data were generated? There would be a standard answer to these questions using the APC multiple-classification specification, if that model were identified. In that case OLS regression or Poisson regression would produce the most likely "generating parameters" based on the data. The problem is that an infinite number of solutions fit the data equally well in the rank deficient by one case.

A constrained solution based on the constraint c_1 is biased to the extent that $E(b_{c1}^0)$ does not equal β. Here b_{c1}^0 is the solution vector under the constraint c_1, E is the expected value operator, and β is the vector of generating parameters. These will only be equal if $c_1'E(b_{c1}^0) = c_1'\beta$; that is, the parameter vector and the expected value of the estimated solution vector under a constraint are each orthogonal to the constraint. In order to provide an unbiased estimate of the generating parameters "all we need to do is find the correct constraint" (c_1). For example, if for the generating parameters age 1 = age 2 and the constraint $(0, 1, -1, 0, 0, \ldots, 0)'$ is used, then $c_1'E(b_{c1}^0)$ will be equal to $c_1'\beta$ and the estimated solution vector would be unbiased. If the constraint is right, all of the rest of the solution is correct in terms of being unbiased. In the third sentence of this paragraph I wrote "all we need to do is find" in quotations, because this is a very difficult task. This requires much more than the solution having strong statistical properties.

All of the constrained solutions provide "best fitting" solutions. The crucial question, however, is whether the constraint is correct or at the very least nearly so. We know that the differences between solutions can be characterized by sv. Kupper et al. (1983) capitalize on this when they suggest the following measure to characterize the degree of bias in a measure [my notation]: $Bias(b_{c1}^0) = sv$, where $s = -c_1'\beta/v'c_1$.[*] Note that the sign of s depends on the coding of the null vector, which is unique only up to multiplication by a scalar, so this is the absolute degree of the bias. We might read this formula as the bias of a solution under the constraint c_1 is sv where s is defined as in the preceding sentence. Kupper et al. (1983:2796) note [my notation]: "Thus, the 'amount' of bias attendant with the use of constraint $c_1'b_{c1}^0 = 0$ depends essentially on how 'close' the corresponding population linear function $c_1'\beta$ is to zero; in particular, there is no bias if c_1 is orthogonal to the (unknown) parameter vector β."

Importantly, Kupper et al. (1983) note that bias is much more important in the context of APC models than the variance associated with the standard errors of the APC model coefficients. They note this smaller variance property for the estimator that is orthogonal to the null vector (the IE before it had a name), and state: "Of course, when the squared multiple correlation coefficient R^2 is fairly close to 1, a result which seems to occur not infrequently in practice, then bias becomes the main area of concern" (p. 2797). Kupper et al.'s point is noteworthy: statistical properties of a constrained estimator

---

[*] This expression for s can be derived from the line of solutions: $b_c^0 = b_{c1}^0 + sv$. Note that β is one of the solutions on the line of solutions, so we can write $\beta = b_{c1}^0 + sv$. Multiplying the equation through by the constraint c_1' yields $c_1'\beta = c_1'b_{c1}^0 + c_1'sv$. Since a solution is orthogonal to *its* constraint, the first term on the right-hand side of the equation is zero leaving $c_1'\beta = c_1'sv$ and $s = c_1'\beta/c_1'v$. Note that $v'c_1 = c_1'v$, they are both dot products, and the sign of s depends on the coding of the null vector, which is unique up to multiplication of a scalar. Thus, $s = c_1'\beta/v'c_1$, where depending on the coding of v, s may be positive or negative.

such as the variance of coefficient estimates is important, but bias is almost certain to be much more important when considering APC models.[*]

I am insistent that there is no mechanical solution for the APC model that results in unbiased estimates of the parameters that generated the outcome variable. One reason for this insistence is that there has been some confusion about whether the IE (or partial least squares or using the Moore–Penrose generalized inverse or principal components analysis) provides an unbiased estimate in the sense of unbiased estimates of the parameters that generated the outcome data. These estimates do not provide such estimates. If any of these methods did provide such an unbiased solution, they would be solutions to the identification problem for rank deficient by one matrix. The sense in which the IE and other constrained estimates are unbiased estimates is made clear in the next section.

2.12 Unbiased Estimation under a Constraint

We can use the term *unbiased* in another sense, one that does not consider the closeness of the expected value of the constrained solution to the data generating parameters. In this sense, constrained estimates are unbiased estimates under the particular constraint employed. That is, they are unbiased estimates of the population parameters associated with the constraint. This sense of unbiasedness applies to the traditional constrained estimates such as setting the first two age coefficients to be equal or the first two period coefficients to be equal, as well as to other constrained estimators such as the IE (principal components analysis and using the Moore–Penrose generalized inverse). Fu, Land, and Yang (2011:457) state that "the IE is not b [the vector of generating parameters β] but rather the projection of b onto the non-null vector space spanned by the column vectors of the design matrix X of the accounting model denoted by b_0 [the intrinsic estimator]." As they note "the IE is not b [the vector of generating parameters β]." It is not an unbiased estimate of β. Using my terminology, the IE is not an unbiased estimate of the parameters that generated the outcome values. The intrinsic estimator is an unbiased estimate of the parameters associated with the constraint that makes the solution vector orthogonal to the null vector.

We can project the generating parameter vector to any of the constrained solution vectors in the following manner: $b_{c1}^0 = G_{c1}\beta$. Here G_{c1} is the generalized inverse associated with the constrained solution b_{c1}^0. Any of the

---

[*] Yang, Fu, and Land (2004:102) note: "For any finite number p of time periods, the intrinsic estimator B has a variance smaller than that of any [other constrained estimators]—i.e., var($\hat{b}$) – var(B) is positive-definite for a nontrivial identifying constraint." Nontrivial here is in the sense that the constraint isn't the same as the constraint associated with the IE or one that produces the IE.

constrained solutions are linear functions of the generating parameters. In fact we can project any solution on the line of solutions to a particular constrained estimate: $b_{c1}^0 = G_{c1} b_c^0$. Any solution on the line of solutions is a linear function of the other solutions on the line of solutions. In terms of these properties there is nothing special about any one of the constrained solutions. I prove the unbiasedness of constrained estimates under their constraint in Appendix 2.3.

2.13 A Plausible Constraint with Some Extra Empirical Support

The obvious task when using the constrained regression approach to the APC identification problem is getting the constraint right. Finding a single constraint that agrees with the data generating parameters produces a constrained estimate that is an unbiased estimate of these underlying parameters. Setting a constraint that approximately agrees with the parameters that generated the data produces somewhat biased estimates. The data for this example appear in Table 2.10 and are drawn from O'Brien et al. (2000). In this age–period table the age categories are 15–19, 20–24, ..., 45–49. The periods are single years spaced 5 years apart: 1960, 1965, ..., 1995. The data were drawn from the Uniform Crime Reports for these years and that source used aggregated 5-year age categories to report most of the arrest rates for homicide offending. The periods and age groups used in Table 2.10 imply the cohorts of interest which range from the earliest cohort born between 1910 and 1914, and the most recent born between 1975 and 1979. As noted

TABLE 2.10

Age–Period-Specific Homicide Arrest Rates (per 100,000) in the United States: 1960 to 1995

Age Group	Period							
	1960	1965	1970	1975	1980	1985	1990	1995
15–19	8.98	9.07	17.22	17.54	18.02	16.32	36.52	35.34
20–24	14	15.18	23.76	25.62	23.95	21.11	29.1	32.34
25–29	13.45	14.69	20.09	21.05	18.91	16.79	17.99	16.75
30–34	10.73	11.7	16	15.81	15.22	12.59	12.44	10.05
35–39	9.37	9.76	13.13	12.83	12.31	9.6	9.38	7.27
40–44	6.48	7.41	10.1	10.52	8.79	7.5	6.81	5.48
45–49	5.71	5.56	7.51	7.32	6.76	5.31	5.17	3.67

Source: Data are from O'Brien (2000), who obtained these data from the Uniform Crime Reports for the years corresponding to these periods. More detail is available in O'Brien (2000).

earlier in Chapter 1, these cohorts do not exactly correspond to the people of these ages in these years, but this makes no difference in the identification problem.

The constraint utilized is a zero linear trend (ZLT) constraint on the period coefficients. That is, the period effects in the solution have a trend of zero. This constraint can be implemented using the Mazumdar et al. (1980) procedure by replacing the last row of $X'X$ with zeros except for the columns of that row corresponding to the periods that are coded from the earliest to the most recent period as − 7, −6, −5, …, −1. We then proceed with the remainder of Mazumdar et al.'s procedure. This constraint forces this trend to be zero and identifies the model.[*]

To the extent that the generating period effect parameters over this series of periods have little or no trend, the results of this analysis will not be too biased. I justify this constraint on the basis of a comprehensive analysis of violent crime rates over time and their relationship to one another (O'Brien et al. 2003) and the justification in O'Brien (2011). Even if we accept the research and logic of O'Brien et al. as providing theoretical/substantive backing for using the zero linear trend for period constraint, I would suggest "methodological modesty" when reporting the results of an APC analysis based on this constraint. The constraint is plausible as an approximation but may be wrong; we saw in Figure 2.1 how getting the trend wrong can result in substantially different results (a rotation of solutions). In Chapter 7 I use several of the methods covered in this book to return to this substantive problem in a more comprehensive manner.

The results of the zero linear trend in period analysis appear in Figure 2.3. The trend in the period effects, panel (b), has been set by the constraint: there is no overall trend in the period coefficients. The rate of increase in homicide offending is greatest from 1960 to 1970 and this fits with the creation of the President's Commission on Law Enforcement and the Administration of Justice and the establishment of the Law Enforcement Assistance Administration (LEAA) that began operations in the late 1960s. O'Brien (2003) suggests that this was a direct response to a real and substantial increase in violent crime. Criminologists also argue that there has been a real and substantial drop in violent crime that occurred after 1990 (Levitt 2004; Zimring 2007). This drop is evident in Figure 2.3b. The age curve for the age effects in panel (a), which is based on the period constraint, is consistent with the "invariant" homicide age curve. Criminologists generally expect the peak of homicide offending to occur in the 20–24 age group followed by the 25–29 age group and then the 15–19 age group with a monotonic decrease in rates after

---

[*] To be explicit, it is better to say that "the model is identified under the constraint." Mason et al. (1973:248) state that "age, cohort and period effects are estimable under the assumption that two coefficients are equal within one of the three dimensions." But as we note in Chapter 4, "estimable" in this sense of being identified under a single constraint is not the same as an estimable function that produces the same results no matter what the constraint.

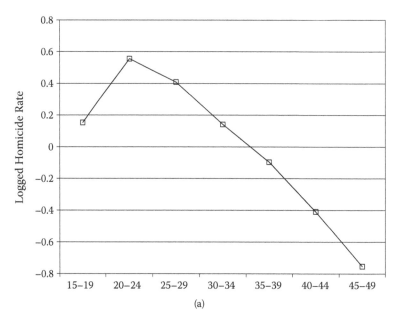

FIGURE 2.3
Plot of estimated age, period, and cohort effects for homicide arrest rates identified by using a ZLT constraint for periods. (a) Age effects, (b) period effects, (c) cohort effects. *(continued)*

the 20–24 age group (Eisner 2003; Hirschi and Gottfredson 1983). The ZLT in period constraint produces a quite plausible age curve. The cohort effects curve is the one for which there is little knowledge/consensus in criminology, but it fits the conjectures and evidence in O'Brien, Stockard, and Isaacson (1999), who argue that the epidemic of youth homicide that occurred in the late 1980s to mid-1990s was a product of increased homicide proneness of cohorts. This is consistent with the steep increase in the cohort effects for the last two cohorts in panel (c). The relative flatness of the cohort effects for the remaining cohorts is consistent with the relative stability of the observed age distribution of homicide offending from 1965 to 1985.

The plausibility of the age curve and the cohort curve add to our confidence in the constraint used to produce these results: the zero linear trend in periods constraint. Although such plausible relationships should build confidence, authors should be modest in their claims based on any constraint used. The results are no better than the constraint and the exact form of the constraint is almost always subject to debate. I have a colleague who is an exceptional quantitative methodologist, and he suggests that reading the result of an APC constrained model is like taking a Rorschach test: you can interpret almost any result in a way that makes sense—at least to you.

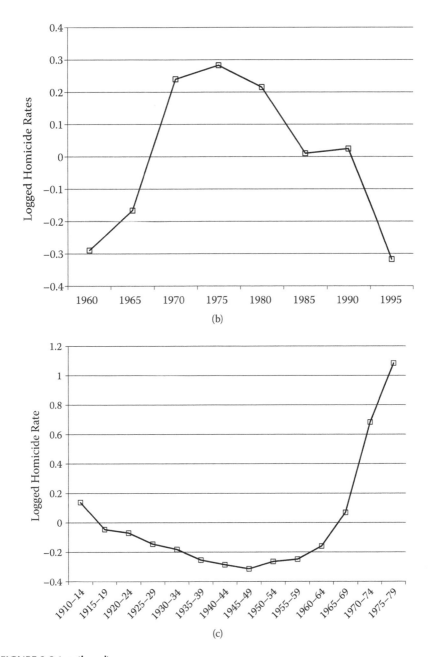

FIGURE 2.3 (continued)
Plot of estimated age, period, and cohort effects for homicide arrest rates identified by using a ZLT constraint for periods. (a) Age effects, (b) period effects, (c) cohort effects.

2.14 Conclusions

Constrained estimation is the most common method used by those seeking to estimate each of the age, period, and cohort coefficients in APC models that use aggregate-level data. Traditionally, constraints in such models have been conceptually simple such as setting two effect coefficients to be equal: for example, age1 = age2 or period2 = period3. Recently, more complex constraints have been introduced; for example, the zero linear trend (which constrains the linear trend in the coefficients of age or period or cohort to be zero), or the intrinsic estimator (which constrains the coefficients in the solution to be orthogonal to the null vector). But in each of these cases these constraints just identify the model and like other constraints need to be justified on the basis of research or theory.

These constrained solutions share many similarities. Each of them just identifies the APC model that otherwise is rank deficient by one, and they fit the data equally well. We cannot use data fit to adjudicate which set of estimates best represents the underlying "true" data generating parameters. This lack of a unique best fitting model is a crucial problem, because conventionally the "best fit criterion" is used to determine the solution that best represents the underlying parameters. If we decide to use one of the constrained solutions as the best representative of parameters that generated the outcome data, we need to justify this choice based on substantive/theoretical criteria and need to be very cautious in our conclusions.

Although fit cannot be used to decide between the various constrained solutions, we do know that all of the constrained solutions are "best fitting" models: they are least squares solutions in the OLS regression context or maximum likelihood estimates in the generalized linear model context. All of the constrained solutions lie on a line that I label the line of solutions: $b_c^0 = b_{c1}^0 + sv$. This shows us how all of the constrained solutions are related to one another and allows for the derivation of a definition of bias in terms of estimating the data generating parameters: $Bias(b_{c1}^0) = sv$, where $s = -c_1'\beta/v'c_1$. Two other shared characteristics of constrained solutions are that the solution is orthogonal to the constraint used to determine the solution and that each of the constrained solutions is an unbiased solution under the constraint (not surprising given the model is just identified under the constraint).

This chapter represents a relatively thorough introduction to *aggregate-level constrained APC models*. These models represent the most commonly used approaches to analyzing aggregate-level APC data. Other topics central to the literature addressing aggregate-level APC analyses for aggregate-level data are covered in later chapters. Before moving to those approaches, the next chapter examines the geometry of APC models.

Appendix 2.1: Dummy Variable and Effect Coding

Dummy Variable Coding for the X-Matrix Based on a 4×4 Age–Period Table

Intercept	age1	age2	age3	per1	per2	per3	coh1	coh2	coh3	coh4	coh5	coh6
1	1	0	0	1	0	0	0	0	0	1	0	0
1	0	1	0	1	0	0	0	0	1	0	0	0
1	0	0	1	1	0	0	0	1	0	0	0	0
1	0	0	0	1	0	0	1	0	0	0	0	0
1	1	0	0	0	1	0	0	0	0	0	1	0
1	0	1	0	0	1	0	0	0	0	1	0	0
1	0	0	1	0	1	0	0	0	1	0	0	0
1	0	0	0	0	1	0	0	1	0	0	0	0
1	1	0	0	0	0	1	0	0	0	0	0	1
1	0	1	0	0	0	1	0	0	0	0	1	0
1	0	0	1	0	0	1	0	0	0	1	0	0
1	0	0	0	0	0	1	0	0	1	0	0	0
1	1	0	0	0	0	0	0	0	0	0	0	0
1	0	1	0	0	0	0	0	0	0	0	0	1
1	0	0	1	0	0	0	0	0	0	0	1	0
1	0	0	0	0	0	0	0	0	0	1	0	0

Effect Coding for the X-Matrix Based on a 4×4 Age–Period Table

intercept	age1	age2	age3	per1	per2	per3	coh1	coh2	coh3	coh4	coh5	coh6
1	1	0	0	1	0	0	0	0	0	1	0	0
1	0	1	0	1	0	0	0	0	1	0	0	0
1	0	0	1	1	0	0	0	1	0	0	0	0
1	−1	−1	−1	1	0	0	1	0	0	0	0	0
1	1	0	0	0	1	0	0	0	0	0	1	0
1	0	1	0	0	1	0	0	0	0	1	0	0
1	0	0	1	0	1	0	0	0	1	0	0	0
1	−1	−1	−1	0	1	0	0	1	0	0	0	0
1	1	0	0	0	0	1	0	0	0	0	0	1
1	0	1	0	0	0	1	0	0	0	0	1	0
1	0	0	1	0	0	1	0	0	0	1	0	0
1	−1	−1	−1	0	0	1	0	0	1	0	0	0
1	1	0	0	−1	−1	−1	−1	−1	−1	−1	−1	−1
1	0	1	0	−1	−1	−1	0	0	0	0	0	1
1	0	0	1	−1	−1	−1	0	0	0	0	1	0
1	−1	−1	−1	−1	−1	−1	0	0	0	1	0	0

Appendix 2.2: Determining Null Vectors for Effect and Dummy Variable Coded Variables

Kupper et al. (1985) provide a formula to find the null vector when effect coding is used and their formula (our notation) is convenient:

$$0, \sum_{i=1}^{I-1}\left[i-\frac{(I+1)}{2}\right]A_i - \sum_{j=1}^{J-1}\left[j-\frac{(J+1)}{2}\right]P_j + \sum_{k=1}^{I+J-2}\left[k-\frac{(I+K)}{2}\right]C_k = 0. \quad (A2.2.1)$$

The first zero is for the intercept. A_i represents the columns of X that correspond to the age effect variables, P_j represents the columns of X that correspond to the period effect variables, and C_k represents the columns of X that correspond to the cohort effect variables. The elements of the null vector for the age, period, and cohort effects are within the square brackets in Equation (A2.2.1), where I, J, and K are the number of ages, periods, and cohorts, respectively. As an example of using Equation (A2.2.1), with a 4 × 4 age–period matrix, the null vector elements for age are –1.5, –.5, and .5. For period they are 1.5, .5, and –.5. For cohorts the null vector elements are –3, –2, –1, 0, 1, and 2. Note that the minus sign in front of the summation symbol for periods makes the numbers within the square brackets change signs. The entire Equation (A2.2.1) is meant to show that the sum of the null vector elements times their corresponding columns results in a column of zeros; that is, $Xv = 0$. As shown in this chapter, the null vector is helpful in understanding the solutions using constrained regression.

It is possible to determine the null vector when dummy variable coding is used. In this case X is the design matrix for dummy variable coding. The formula for finding the null vector (using the oldest age group, most recent period, and most recent cohort as reference groups) is

$$\text{int}, \sum_{i=1}^{I-1}[i-I]A_i - \sum_{j=1}^{J-1}[j-J]P_j + \sum_{k=1}^{I+J-2}\left[k-(I+J-1)\right]C_k = 0 \quad (A2.2.2)$$

Here, A_i, P_j, C_k, I, J, and K are defined as in Equation (A2.2.1), except that the A_i, P_j, and C_k columns are coded as dummy variables. The intercept element of the null vector (int), however, is not zero. We can find it by noting the following relationship: intercept $+ v_{ia} + v_{jp} + v_{kc} = 0$, where $k = I - i + j$, v_{ia} equals the ith age element of the null vector, v_{jp} equals the jth period element of the null vector, and v_{kc} equals the $(I - i + j)$th cohort element of the null vector:

$$\text{intercept} = -(v_{ia} + v_{jp} + v_{kc}). \quad (A2.2.3)$$

We can always check whether we have correctly calculated the null vector by making sure that $Xv = 0$.

As an example, for a 4×4 age–period matrix the null vector elements for age are -3, -2, and -1. For period they are $+3$, $+2$, and $+1$. For cohorts the null vector elements are -6, -5, -4, -3, -2, and -1. When we put these elements into the null vector and add a $+3$ as the first element for the intercept, these elements times the columns of the dummy variable coded X matrix produce a zero vector of 13 elements or in the notation introduced earlier $Xv = 0$. We calculated the intercept using Equation (A2.2.3). If we take the second age group in the second period in order to calculate the intercept, we find that $v_{2a} = -2$, $v_{2p} = +2$, and $v_{4c} = -3$ (v_{4c} is the null element of the cohort corresponding to the second age group in the second period). The intercept equals $3 \ [= -(- 2+2-3)]$.

The generalization is straightforward. In a 5×3 age–period matrix with dummy variable coding, the null vector elements for age are -4, -3, -2, and -1, for period they are 2 and 1, and for cohort they are -6, -5, -4, -3 -2, and -1. The intercept based on the youngest age group in the first period and the fifth cohort (which corresponds to being in the youngest age group in the first period) is determined as follows: $v_{1a} = -4$, $v_{1p} = 2$, and $v_{5c} = -2$ and the intercept equals $4 \ [= - (-4 + 2 - 2)]$.

Appendix 2.3 Constrained Estimates as Unbiased Estimates

By definition the constrained population parameter β_{c1} is orthogonal to the constraint c_1: $c_1'\beta_{c1} = 0$. To show that the constrained estimate is an unbiased estimate of β_{c1}, I show that its expected value is orthogonal to c_1. To solve for b_{c1}^0 I write the matrix equation $y = Xb_{c1} + \epsilon$. Multiplying this matrix equation through by the transpose of X yields

$$X'y = X'Xb_{c1}^0 + X'\epsilon. \tag{A2.3.1}$$

To solve for b_{c1}^0 a generalized inverse based on the c_1 constraint is used to premultiply the equation above by this generalized inverse. The result is

$$(X'X)_{c1}^- X'y = (X'X)_{c1}^- X'Xb_{c1}^0 + (X'X)_{c1}^- X'\epsilon. \tag{A2.3.2}$$

Taking expectations $(X'X)_{c1}^- X'y = E(b_{c1}^0)$, since $E(X'\epsilon) = 0$. Since this estimate is under the constraint c_1: $c_1'E(b_{c1}^0) = 0$.) Therefore, $c_1'E_1(b_{c1}^0) = c_1'\beta_{c1}$ and $E(b_{c1}^0) = \beta_{c1}$. This constrained estimator is an unbiased estimate of the constrained parameters.

References

Clayton, D., and E. Schifflers. 1987. Models for temporal variation in cancer rates II: Age-period-cohort models. *Statistics in Medicine* 6:468–81.

Eisner, M. 2003. Long term historical trends in violent crime. *Crime & Justice: A Review of Research* 30: 83–142.

Fienberg, S.E., and W.M. Mason. 1979. Identification and estimation of age-period-cohort models in the analysis of discrete archival data. *Sociological Methodology* 10:1–67.

Greene, W.H. 1993. *Econometric Analysis* (2nd edition). New York: MacMillan.

Hirschi, T., and M.R. Gottfredson. 1983. Age and the explanation of crime. *American Journal of Sociology* 89:552–84.

Kupper, L.L., J.M. Janis, I.A. Salama, C.N. Yoshizawa, and B.G. Greenberg. 1983. Age-period-cohort analysis: An illustration of the problems in assessing interaction in one observation per cell data. *Communications in Statistics* 12:2779–807.

Kupper, L.L., J.M. Janis, A. Karmous, and B.G. Greenberg. 1985. Statistical age-period-cohort analysis: A review and critique. *Journal of Chronic Disease* 38:811–30.

Levitt, S.D. 2004. Understanding why crime fell in the 1990s: Four factors that explain the decline and six that do not. *Journal of Economic Perspectives* 18: 163–90.

Mason, K.O., W.M. Mason, H.H. Winsborough, and W.K. Poole. 1973. Some methodological issues in cohort analysis of archival data. *American Sociological Review* 38:242–58.

Mason, W.M., and S.E. Fienberg (eds.). 1985. *Cohort Analysis in Social Research: Beyond the Identification Approach*. New York: Springer-Verlag.

Mazumdar, S., C.C. Li, and G.R. Bryce. 1980. Correspondence between a linear restriction and a generalized inverse in linear model analysis. *The American Statistician* 34:103–05.

McCullagh, P., and J.A. Nelder. 1989. *Generalized Linear Models* (2nd edition). New York: Chapman & Hall.

O'Brien, R.M. 2003. UCR violent crime rates, 1958–2000: Recorded and offender-generated trends. *Social Science Research* 32:499–518.

O'Brien, R.M. 2011. Constrained estimators and age-period-cohort models. *Sociological Methods & Research* 40:419–52.

O'Brien, R.M., J. Stockard, and L. Isaacson. 1999. The enduring effects of cohort size and percent of nonmarital births on age-specific homicide rates, 1960–1995. *American Journal of Sociology* 104:1061–95.

Scheffé, H. 1959. *The Analysis of Variance*. New York: John Wiley & Sons.

Searle, S.R. 1971. *Linear Models*. New York: John Wiley & Sons.

Yang, Y., W.J. Fu, and K.C. Land. 2004. A methodological comparison of age-period-cohort models: Intrinsic estimator and conventional generalized linear models. In *Sociological Methodology*, ed. R.M. Stolzenberg, 75–110. Oxford: Basil Blackwell.

Yang, Y., and K.C. Land. 2013a. *Age-Period-Cohort Analysis: New Models, Methods, and Empirical Applications*. New York: Chapman & Hall.

Yang, Y., and K.C. Land. 2013b. Misunderstandings, mischaracterizations, and the problematic choice of a specific instance in which the IE should never be applied. *Demography*, 50:1969–71.

Zimring, F.E. 2007. *The Great American Crime Decline*. New York: Oxford University Press.

3

Geometry of Age–Period–Cohort (APC) Models and Constrained Estimation

> As long as algebra and geometry have been separated, their progress has been slow and their uses limited; but when these two sciences have been united, they have lent each mutual force, and have marched together towards perfection.
>
> **Joseph Louis Lagrange, 1795**

3.1 Introduction

Conceiving of statistical problems visually can be a great aid to understanding. Ronald Fisher used this method to develop many novel tests and statistical procedures. He was noted for seeing relationships geometrically and notorious for not proving them algebraically until sometimes much later (Box 1978:122–9). A basic understanding of the geometry of age–period–cohort (APC) models enhances understanding of the APC identification problem and the different approaches used to "solve" those models.

This chapter presents a geometry of the APC identification problem. This geometry is presented from a "row perspective." It takes each row of the normal equations as a geometric object in an m-dimensional solution space rather than taking a "column perspective" and examining each column (Strang 1998). In classic APC models the matrix of independent variables is one less than full column rank. This is true whether considering age, period, and cohort to be measured continuously on an interval level (age in years of age, period in year by date, and cohorts in year of birth) or as categorical variables using dummy variable or effect coding for the categories of age, period, and cohort. Since we are dealing with APC models, the focus is on the geometry of the rank deficient by one model and how, from a geometric perspective, constrained solutions work.[*]

---

[*] O'Brien (2012) discusses the rank deficient by one situation and situations of greater rank deficiency, and some parts of this chapter are derived from that article.

The simplest multiple equation system (without reference to APC models) that takes the row perspective shows clearly the problem of linear dependency. To facilitate the development of this perspective, I address the case of just one independent variable (one dimension) and then move to two and three dimensions (two or three independent variables). This approach is extended to the *m*-dimensional case. The geometric perspective clarifies how constrained regression addresses the problems introduced by the rank deficient by one case. The focus then shifts explicitly to APC models. In this more specific substantive context, the readers are invited to think about how much confidence they have in any one of these particular solutions and what would give them added confidence in the solution provided by any particular constrained solution. The discussion ends with some of the insights into APC models that can be gained from this geometric perspective.

3.2 General Geometric View of Rank Deficient by One Models

I begin by examining the normal equations and their hyperplane representations. The emphasis is on the intersection of these hyperplanes and the fact that in the rank deficient by one situation one of the hyperplanes does not intersect (in a point) the line formed by the intersection of all of the other hyperplanes. The setting is an *m*-dimensional solution space. Pedagogically, it makes sense to begin with one, two, and three dimensions to build an intuitive bridge to the geometry of the rank deficient by one model in the general case of *m*-dimensions. The problem, as we will see, is that although $m - 1$ of the hyperplanes (representing $m - 1$ of the normal equations) intersect one another to form a line in the *m*-dimensional solution space, the remaining hyperplane (representing the remaining normal equation) does not intersect this line in a point; instead the line lies on the surface of this remaining hyperplane.

This geometry applies to any rank deficient by one situation. For example, in addition to the APC case this rank deficient by one situation occurs when

1. The total test score consists of the score on the math section plus the score on the verbal section and one wants to assess the independent effects of the total score (TS), the math score (MS), and the verbal score (VS) on college GPA. The linear dependency is VS + MS = TS.
2. Separating the effects of educational status (ES), occupational status (OS), and status inconsistency (SI): SI = OS − ES (Blalock 1967).
3. Disentangling the effects of origin status (OrigS), destination status (DS), and the degree of mobility DM: DM = DS − OrigS (Duncan 1966).
4. For the linear coding of the APC model: P − A = C.

The linear dependency is more complex in the APC categorically coded situation. For example, the X-matrix postmultiplied by the null vector for the 5×5 age–period table, can be written as $\mathbf{0} = X(0, -2, -1, 0, 1, \ldots, 2, 3)'$ (see Chapter 2, Appendix 2.2). This means that the dot product of the null vector elements and each of the rows of the matrix of independent variables equals zero: $Xv = \mathbf{0}$. One way to write this linear dependency in terms of one of the independent variables being linearly dependent upon the other independent variables is $a_1 = 0.00 \times \text{intercept} - .50a_2 + 0.00a_3 + .50a_4 + \ldots + 1.00c_7 + 1.50c_8$. That is, the values of a_1 can be perfectly determined from the values of the other independent variables.

The normal equations associated with ordinary least squares (OLS) regression will be used throughout, since this is the situation most familiar to readers. But the geometry with generalized linear models is equivalent, given that in those models the dependent variables are linear functions of the independent variables (see Chapter 2). Beginning with the simplest situation, the bivariate case, the mean of the independent variable is subtracted from each independent variable score and the mean of the dependent variable is subtracted from each dependent variable score. This creates deviation scores and allows us to concentrate on the regression coefficient between these two variables, since the intercept is zero.

As is well known, in the one independent–one dependent variable situation, there are only two quantities needed to find the slope: the sums of squares for the independent variable (Σx^2) and the sum of products for the independent and dependent variables (Σxy). In this two-variable situation using deviation scores there is one normal equation

$$\left(\sum x^2 \right) b = \sum xy, \tag{3.1}$$

yielding the well-known solution $b = \Sigma xy / \Sigma x^2$. Using matrix algebra, we write Equation (3.1) as $X'Xb = X'y$, where X is a $n \times 1$ vector of the independent variable deviations, and y is an $n \times 1$ vector of the y deviations on the dependent variable. The prime means that the column vector has been transposed (in this case into a row vector). Carrying out the matrix multiplications yields a single equation: Equation (3.1). For concreteness, values for Σx^2 and Σxy were created: $\Sigma x^2 = 4$ and $\Sigma xy = 8$. Then Equation (3.1) can be written as $4b = 8$ and $b = 2$. Geometrically, the solution space has only one dimension (b) and Equation (3.1) represents a unique point on this line. Solving the equation determines where on that one dimension of possible values for b the solution lies.

In the situation of two independent variables, we again center the variables by subtracting their means from their raw scores so that all of the variables are in deviation score form. The two independent variables are distinguished by subscripting them with a one or a two: x_1 or x_2.

From an algebraic perspective the quantities of interest are Σx_1^2, Σx_2^2, $\Sigma x_1 x_2$, $\Sigma x_1 y$ and $\Sigma x_2 y$. Formulas that appear in a number of introductory texts covering multiple regression allow one to place these quantities into formulas and solve for the two regression coefficients (Cohen, Cohen, West, and Aiken 2003; Fox 2008). The matrix algebra representation remains the same $X'Xb = X'y$, but now the X-matrix contains two columns (one for each of the independent variables) and n rows (one for each of the observations). The vector b has two elements: one for the regression coefficient for the first independent variable (b_1) and one for the second independent variable (b_2). The explicit matrix form of the equations using the sums of squares and cross-products (remembering all of the variables are in deviation score form) is

$$\begin{bmatrix} \sum x_1^2 & \sum x_1 x_2 \\ \sum x_2 x_1 & \sum x_2^2 \end{bmatrix} \begin{bmatrix} b_1 \\ b_2 \end{bmatrix} = \begin{bmatrix} \sum x_1 y \\ \sum x_2 y \end{bmatrix}. \tag{3.2}$$

Carrying out the matrix multiplication in Equation (3.2), the two normal equations are

$$\left(\sum x_1^2 \right) b_1 + \left(\sum x_1 x_2 \right) b_2 = \sum x_1 y$$
$$\left(\sum x_2 x_1 \right) b_1 + \left(\sum x_2^2 \right) b_2 = \sum x_2 y \tag{3.3}$$

Each of these is the equation for a line (the general form of the equation for a line is ($Ab_1 + Bb_2 = c$). We again supply some appropriate values for the sums of squares and cross-products [Σx_1^2, Σx_2^2, $\Sigma x_1 x_2$, $\Sigma x_1 y$, and $\Sigma x_2 y$] and placing these into Equation (3.3) produces a set of two normal equations that could result from real data,

$$4b_1 + 2b_2 = 8$$
$$2b_1 - 3b_2 = -4. \tag{3.4}$$

We can solve this two-equation system by, for example, substituting $1.5b_2 - 2$ (derived from the second equation) into the first equation for b_1; we find that $b_2 = 2$ and then knowing b_2 we can easily solve for b_1, which is equal to 1.

Geometrically, the solution space now has two dimensions: one for b_1 and one for b_2. The normal equations in (3.4) are equations for lines, and if these two lines intersect at a point in this two-dimensional solution space, they determine a unique solution to this two-equation system. This is depicted in Figure 3.1. The horizontal axis represents the b_1 dimension and the vertical

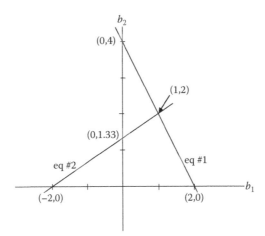

FIGURE 3.1
Solution for the two independent variable situation in Equation (3.4).

line the b_2 dimension. We construct the two lines based on the equations in Equation (3.4) in the following manner. Using the first equation in (3.4): if $b_2 = 0$ then $b_1 = 2$, so that one of the points on the line is (2, 0). Similarly, if $b_1 = 0$ then $b_2 = 4$, and a second point on this first line is (0, 4) and these two points allow us to draw this first line (the line for equation one) in the two-dimensional solution space. The second line is constructed in the same manner, if we set $b_2 = 0$ then $b_1 = -2$, so one point on the line is (-2, 0). If we set $b_1 = 0$ then $b_2 = 1.33$, then a second point on the second line is (0, 1.33). This allows us to construct the second line. These two lines intersect at (1, 2) that is $b_1 = 1$ and $b_2 = 2$. This is the geometric view of the solution to the normal equations with two independent variables. It is likely familiar to most readers.

Imagine the situation in which the two equations are linearly dependent, for example,

$$4b_1 + 2b_2 = 8$$
$$2b_1 + 1b_2 = 4.$$

(3.5)

The second equation is one-half times the first equation. There is no unique solution to these equations. When we substitute the second equations value for b_1 (= $-.50b_2 + 2$) into the first equation's value for b_1 and solve for b_2, we obtain $0b_2 = 0$. This is a rather uninformative result, since b_2 could take on any value. The value of b_2 is not identified. If we substitute the second equation value for b_2 into the first equation, we find that $0b_1 = 0$. Geometrically we can plot the first equation as before and end up with the line for the first equation in Figure 3.1. When we plot the line representing the second equation, we find that it also crosses the b_1 axis at (2, 0) and the b_2 axis at (0, 4). That is, the lines for these two equations are coincident; they lie on each other. Any solutions to these equations lie on this line. For example, (2, 0) is a solution to both of these equations, as are (0, 4) and (1, 2). There are an infinite number of solutions to these two equations and they all lie on this line in a solution space of two dimensions.

One informative way to write the equation for this line is as the "vector equation for a line," that is, as one of the points on the line plus a scalar (s) times the "direction of the line":

$$\begin{bmatrix} 0 \\ 4 \end{bmatrix} + s \begin{bmatrix} 1 \\ -2 \end{bmatrix}.$$

The direction is one over to the right on b_1 and two down on b_2. To show how this formula works, note that it previously has been shown that (0, 4) is on this line, and it is the solution when $s = 0$; (1, 2) is on this line, and it is the solution when $s = 1$; and (2, 0) is on this line, and it is the solution when $s = 2$. Selecting other values for s will produce the other points on this line; that is, any of the other solutions to this set of two equations. Importantly, although there are an infinite number of solutions to this set of two equations, the only solutions are those that lie on this line.

The null vector is the vector that when postmultiplied times a matrix results in a vector of zeros. In the normal equations context, the null vector is the vector (not consisting of all zeros) that when premultiplied by $X'X$ produces a vector of zeros. Writing the $X'X$-matrix for Equation (3.5), we have

$$\begin{bmatrix} 4 & 2 \\ 2 & 1 \end{bmatrix}$$

and note that the vector

$$\begin{bmatrix} 1 \\ -2 \end{bmatrix}$$

when premultiplied by $X'X$ produces the vector

$$\begin{bmatrix} 0 \\ 0 \end{bmatrix}.$$

The null vector for this matrix is $(1, -2)'$ and is represented as v. It is unique up to multiplication by a scalar. There is only one null vector for Equation (3.5), because there is only one linear dependency. Note that the line of solutions is parallel to the null vector, since they share the same direction. The null vector is represented as a line running through the $(0, 0)$ point with a slope of -2.

The most complex situation in which the solutions and the problems caused by the linear dependency among the independent variables can be concretely visualized geometrically is the situation in which there are three independent variables. Following is the explicit matrix equation of sums of squares and cross-products for this three variable situation:

$$\begin{bmatrix} \sum x_1^2 & \sum x_1 x_2 & \sum x_1 x_3 \\ \sum x_2 x_1 & \sum x_2^2 & \sum x_2 x_3 \\ \sum x_3 x_1 & \sum x_3 x_2 & \sum x_3^2 \end{bmatrix} \begin{bmatrix} b_1 \\ b_2 \\ b_3 \end{bmatrix} = \begin{bmatrix} \sum x_1 y \\ \sum x_2 y \\ \sum x_3 y \end{bmatrix} \qquad (3.6)$$

We can write out the three normal equations implied by this matrix formulation as

$$\left(\sum x_1^2 \right) b_1 + \left(\sum x_1 x_2 \right) b_2 + \left(\sum x_1 x_3 \right) b_3 = \sum x_1 y$$

$$\left(\sum x_2 x_1 \right) b_1 + \left(\sum x_2^2 \right) b_2 + \left(\sum x_2 x_3 \right) b_3 = \sum x_2 y$$

$$\left(\sum x_3 x_1 \right) b_1 + \left(\sum x_3 x_2 \right) b_2 + \left(\sum x_3^2 \right) b_3 = \sum x_3 y . \qquad (3.7)$$

These three normal equations, when solved for b_1, b_2, and b_3, provide the least squares solutions. Geometrically each of these equations represents the equation for a plane: $Ab_1 + Bb_2 + Cb_3 = d$, where A, B, C, and d are real numbers. We again can provide some appropriate numbers for these sums of squares and cross-products (in practice, of course, they are derived from observations). This produces three normal equations for the data:

$$4b_1 + 4b_2 + 2b_3 = 8$$

$$4b_1 + 6b_2 + 4b_3 = 10$$

$$2b_1 + 2b_2 + 4b_3 = 12. \qquad (3.8)$$

These equations can be solved by substitution as was done to solve the two-equation system in (3.4) or matrix algebra could be used. The solution set is b_1 = 2.333, b_2 = –1.667, and b_3 = 2.667. This solution set is the unique least squares solution set for this data

We could construct our geometrical figure as before except now the solution space has three dimensions: one for b_1, one for b_2, and one for b_3. Each of the three equations represents a plane and to construct one of the planes we determine where the plane for the first equation crosses the b_1 axis; that is, what is the value of b_1 when b_2 and b_3 are both equal to zero. The answer is that b_1 = 2; one point on this plane is (2, 0, 0). Similarly the plane represented by the equation in the first row crosses the b_2 axis at 2 so a second point on the plane is (0, 2, 0). Finally, the plane crosses the b_3 axis at 4 so that another point on the plane is (0, 0, 4). These three points determine the plane represented by the first equation in this three-space. In the same manner, we can determine the plane for the second row equation by finding where it crosses the three axes (2.50, 0, 0) (0, 1.667, 0), and (0, 0, 2.50), and for the third row equation (6, 0, 0), (0, 6, 0), and (0, 0, 3). Any two of these planes are not linearly dependent; they will intersect one another and intersection will determine a line. Here, the third plane is not linearly dependent on the first two planes, so it will intersect this line at a point, and this point will determine the unique solution for this three-equation problem. With no linear dependency, a line and a plane will intersect in a point in a three-space.

The point of intersection (2.333, –1.667, 2.667) will be the same as the solution using algebraic means. A careful geometer would be able to generate this solution using the intersections of planes. Of course, interest focuses on the visualization/intuition supplied by the geometric perspective, and geometric constructions is not recommended as a means for computing such results. For now, we simply need to visualize two planes intersecting in a line in a three-space (imagine the three-space as a room) and another plane crossing that line. That point of intersection supplies the unique coordinates in a three-space and thus a unique solution for the parameter estimates.

A set of equations with a linear dependency appears in Equation (3.9), where the third row equation is one half the first row equation plus one half the second row equation:

$$4b_1 + 4b_2 + 2b_3 = 8$$

$$4b_1 + 6b_2 + 4b_3 = 10$$

$$4b_1 + 5b_2 + 3b_3 = 9. \tag{3.9}$$

There is no unique solution to this set of equations. If we constructed planes for two of these three equations they would intersect in a line, since any two of these equations do not form a linearly dependent set. This line, however, will not intersect the remaining plane in a point, but will lie on the remaining plane. Therefore, any solution on this line will be a solution to this set of equations. In order for there to be a unique solution the remaining plane would have had to intersect the line formed by the intersection of the other two planes at a single point. We depict such a relationship later in this chapter in Figure 3.2 in the substantive context of an APC model.

For the first two equations in (3.9) the line of their intersection can be described by the following vector equation for the line:

$$
\begin{bmatrix} 1 \\ 1 \\ 0 \end{bmatrix} + s \begin{bmatrix} 1 \\ -2 \\ 2 \end{bmatrix}.
\tag{3.10}
$$

The intersection of the second and third planes can be described by the same line as can the intersection of the first and third planes.

The remaining plane does not help us find a unique solution, since it does not intersect with the line at a single point: all of the points on the line lie on the remaining plane and thus there is not a unique intersection point for the line and the plane. If the plane of the remaining equation were not linearly dependent on the other two equations, its plane would intersect the line established by the first two planes. (In constrained regression the remaining plane is forced to change direction and, thus, provide a unique solution under the constraint.)

The null vector for Equation (3.9) is $(1, -2, 2)'$ since:

$$
\begin{bmatrix} 4 & 4 & 2 \\ 4 & 6 & 4 \\ 4 & 5 & 3 \end{bmatrix} \begin{bmatrix} 1 \\ -2 \\ 2 \end{bmatrix} = \begin{bmatrix} 0 \\ 0 \\ 0 \end{bmatrix}.
\tag{3.11}
$$

The null vector is parallel to the line established by the two intersecting planes. We label the line of intersection as the "line of solutions," since any point on that line solves the set of equations that are rank deficient by one. In the APC case any solution on this line is a least squares solutions for the APC model. In the generalized linear model case any solution on the line of solutions is a best fitting solution. Since generalized linear models have a different functional relationship to the independent variables, each of the generalized linear models (e.g., Poisson regression or logistic regression) will have a different line of solutions.

3.3 Generalization to Systems with More Dimensions

Without linearly dependent equations, we find that in the two-variable situation, with all variables in deviation form, the normal equations consist of two equations for lines and these lines intersect in the two-dimensional solution space and provide a unique solution to the equations. With three independent variables there are three normal equations and each one of them is the equation for a plane. These three planes intersect at a unique point in the three-dimensional solution space providing a unique solution to the equations. Venturing beyond these intuitive two- and three-dimensional cases, the generalization/extension is clear, but the terminology and visualizations are more difficult. With four-independent variables there are four normal equations. Each represents a three-dimension hyperplane (one greater than a two-dimensional plane with three independent variables). If there are no linear dependencies, then these four three-dimensional hyperplanes intersect in a point in the four-dimensional solution space and provide a unique solution. With m independent variables there are m normal equations and each one of them represents an $(m - 1)$-dimensional hyperplane. These m hyperplanes intersect in a point in the m-dimensional solution space and provide a unique solution to this set of m equations.

With a linear dependency in the two-variable case the two lines representing the two normal equations coincide; they do not intersect and any solution on these coinciding lines, "the line of solutions," solves the two normal equations. In the three-independent-variable situation, where the three normal equations represent planes, two of the three planes intersect in a line in the three-dimensional solution space, but the remaining plane does not intersect this line at a unique point, the line of solutions lies on the plane. With four independent variables there are four normal equations. Each equation represents a three-dimensional hyperplane and three of the four hyperplanes intersect in a line. The remaining three-dimensional hyperplane does not intersect this line in a point, but the line lies on this remaining hyperplane. This is impossible to visualize concretely, but the generalization is straightforward as it is in the case of m independent variables. Kendall (1961) provides a more technical basis for these results, but covers only the full rank situation. The rules for the extension to rank deficient by one matrices of m dimension appear in Appendix A3.1, which helps to formalize these extensions. The algebra and the geometry, of course, are consistent. I now move explicitly to a consideration of APC models and in this more substantive discussion, of necessity, will repeat some portions of the discussion from earlier in this chapter. This more substantively oriented example explicitly examines how constrained regression works geometrically.

3.4 APC Model with Linearly Coded Variables

We can picture the APC model in a three-space, if age, period, and cohort are coded as continuous interval-level variables so that each are centered around their means and the dependent variable is centered around its mean. Any two of the three variables are linearly independent. For example, knowing the period does not determine the age group and knowing the date of the cohort's birth does not determine the period. The three variables in the same model, however, are not linearly independent of one another. Knowing the period and the age, for example, determines the birth cohort. In this three-variable situation there is a linear dependency among the three variables while any two of these variables are independent of each other.

There are three normal equations and each equation represents a plane. Two of these planes intersect with each other forming a line and the remaining plane does not intersect this line at a point. Instead the line of solutions lies on the remaining plane. We can determine the line on which the solutions must fall, but the remaining plane (equation) does not intersect this line at a single point.

The constrained regression solution to this dilemma is to set the direction of the "remaining plane" so that it intersects the line on which the solutions must fall. One way to do this is to use a generalized inverse based on a particular constraint (Mazumdar, Li, and Bryce, 1980). This provides *a solution* to the system of equations (under that constraint). One can also use any appropriate generalized inverse and the constraint imposed is then typically implicit.

3.4.1 Age, Period, and Cohort as Continuous Variables: A Concrete Example

The easiest APC constraint to visualize is one using the continuous "interval-level coded" age, period, and cohort variables. This would occur if we coded age as years of age, period as year, and cohort as year of birth. If the data were aggregated in 5-year groups, we could code anyone in the 15–19 age category as 17 and in the 20–24 age category as 22, and so on. The periods might be 1990–1994 coded as 1992 and 1995–1999 coded as 1997, and so on. The cohort values would be based on these linearly coded age and period values (Cohort = Period – Age). Here the constraint often employed by researchers is simply not considering one of these three variables in their analysis. For example, a researcher might study the relationship of age and period to a dependent variable without considering cohort effects.

When considering all three components, the linear dependency in such models arises from the fact that Period – Age = Cohort. The equation in this simple case with aggregate-level data for the APC linear model is

$$y_{ij} = \mu + b_a Age_i + b_p Period_j + b_k Cohort_k + e_{ij}, \tag{3.12}$$

where y_{ij} is the rate associated with the *i*th age group in the *j*th period, μ is the intercept, Age_i is the linearly coded age associated with the *i*th age group, Period$_j$ is the linearly coded period associated with the jth period, Cohort$_k$ is the linearly coded cohort associated with the corresponding age and period, and e_{ij} is the residual associated with ith age and jth period observation. Equation (3.12) can be extended to include other variables such as the unemployment rate for each age group at each period (age–period-specific unemployment rates) and/or age squared. This, typically, will not affect the linear dependency that is between the linearly coded age, period, and cohort variables.[*]

3.4.2 Geometry of Age, Period, and Cohort for Linearly Coded Effects

The geometry of this case is simpler than the geometry for the full categorically coded APC model and provides insights that can be used in more complicated situations. Rodgers (1982:782) notes the relationship between the linear components of the age, period, cohort model as [in my notation]

$$b^0_{ac} = b^0_{ac1} + s$$

$$b^0_{pc} = b^0_{pc1} - s$$

$$b^0_{kc} = b^0_{kc1} + s, \qquad (3.13)$$

where the coefficients on the left-hand side are any of the infinite number of estimated linear effects of age, period, and cohort, respectively. The coefficients represented on the right-hand side of the equation are the linear effects for the coefficients under the constraint $c1$, and s is a scalar. There is a linear relationship between the estimated values of these effects, for example, if s is .50 then b^0_{ac} is .50 greater than the regression coefficient under the $c1$ constraint, b^0_{pc} is .50 less than the regression coefficient under the $c1$ constraint, and b^0_{kc} is .50 greater than the coefficient under the $c1$ constraint. It is helpful to write this set of equations in vector form as

$$b^0_c = b^0_{c1} + sv, \qquad (3.14)$$

or more explicitly as

$$\begin{bmatrix} b^0_{ac} \\ b^0_{pc} \\ b^0_{kc} \end{bmatrix} = \begin{bmatrix} b^0_{ac1} \\ b^0_{pc1} \\ b^0_{kc1} \end{bmatrix} + s \begin{bmatrix} 1 \\ -1 \\ 1 \end{bmatrix}. \qquad (3.15)$$

---

[*] These additional variables could affect the linear dependency, if they were linear combinations of age, period, and cohort themselves.

TABLE 3.1

Illustrative Data from a 4 × 4 Age–Period Table

	Original Data				Deviation Data		
Intercept	Age	Period	Cohort	y	Age	Period	Cohort	y
1	41	2005	1964	7	−1.5	−1.5	0	−4.5
1	42	2005	1963	6	−0.5	−1.5	−1	−5.5
1	43	2005	1962	5	0.5	−1.5	−2	−6.5
1	44	2005	1961	4	1.5	−1.5	−3	−7.5
1	41	2006	1965	11	−1.5	−0.5	1	−0.5
1	42	2006	1964	10	−0.5	−0.5	0	−1.5
1	43	2006	1963	9	0.5	−0.5	−1	−2.5
1	44	2006	1962	8	1.5	−0.5	−2	−3.5
1	41	2007	1966	15	−1.5	0.5	2	3.5
1	42	2007	1965	14	−0.5	0.5	1	2.5
1	43	2007	1964	13	0.5	0.5	0	1.5
1	44	2007	1963	12	1.5	0.5	−1	0.5
1	41	2008	1967	19	−1.5	1.5	3	7.5
1	42	2008	1966	18	−0.5	1.5	2	6.5
1	43	2008	1965	17	0.5	1.5	1	5.5
1	44	2008	1964	16	1.5	1.5	0	4.5

The form of Equation (3.14) is that of the vector equation for a line $b_c^0 = b_{c1}^0 + sv$, where b_c^0 represents any of the "best fitting" solutions, b_{c1}^0 is a specific best fitting solution, s is a scalar, and $v = (1, -1, 1)'$ is the null vector and represents the direction of the line. There is an infinite number of solutions to Equation (3.14), and they all lie on a line $b_c^0 = b_{c1}^0 + sv$ in a three-space. To find this line, we do not need to know the parameters "nature used" to generate the outcome data, because from one perspective the generating parameters are just one of the many solutions that lie on the line of solutions. We only need to calculate *a solution* (b_{c1}^0) to the normal equations and then add sv.

To make these relationships more concrete, I present the same constructed data that were used in Chapter 2 in Table 3.1. If we center these variables on their means, we can produce the deviations in Table 3.1. The age, period, and cohort entries in row one of this deviation data are −1.5, −1.5, 0, which when multiplied by $(1, -1, 1)'$ equals zero. The result is the same for each row of the deviation data in Table 3.1. If we use the original data and add a column of ones for the intercept as the first column of the design matrix, then the null vector is $(0, 1, -1, 1)$. In matrix notation we write $Xv = \mathbf{0}$.

The illustrative data in Table 3.1 were created in such a manner that the age trend is 1 and the period and cohort trends are both 2. For these data there is only a trend, but the process is the same with "messier" data.* Transforming the data to deviations from the mean produces simpler numbers, but more importantly eliminates the intercept and allows the line of solutions to be depicted in a three-space. We work with the deviation data in Table 3.1 and compute the following results for the normal equations (3.16):

$$X'X \qquad\qquad b = X'y$$

$$\begin{bmatrix} 20 & 0 & -20 \\ 0 & 20 & 20 \\ -20 & 20 & 40 \end{bmatrix} \begin{bmatrix} b_a \\ b_p \\ b_k \end{bmatrix} = \begin{bmatrix} -20 \\ 80 \\ 100 \end{bmatrix}. \qquad (3.16)$$

Any solution for the vector b in these equations produces a least squares solution. From a row perspective, there is a clear linear dependency in the $X'X$-matrix, since adding the negative of the first row to the second row results in the third row. From a column perspective, we see that adding the negative of column 1 to column 2 equals column 3.

Figure 3.2 depicts the "line of solutions" for this data and the remaining plane. In the situation with three linearly independent variables, the remaining plane would intersect this line of solutions in a point, but in this case with the linear dependency it does not intersect the line of solutions at a unique point. The solution space has three dimensions: one for the age effect, one for the period effect, and the vertical axis representing the cohort effect. I have labeled these axes b_a, b_p, and b_k, respectively. The null vector (1, −1, 1) is depicted as the dotted line through the origin (0, 0, 0). To draw the line of solutions, I determined the point on the line of solutions that would have a zero effect for periods; that is, where the line of solutions would cross the age–cohort plane. That point is (3, 0, 4). We can check whether this point is on the line of solutions by seeing if it produces correct solutions for the normal equations. If the period coefficient is zero, then for each row of the normal equations in (3.15) this solution set (3, 0, 4) produces the correct $X'y$ value. That is, if period is zero, the age coefficient must be 3 and the cohort coefficient 4. The same procedure can be used to determine at what point the line of solutions crosses the period–cohort plane: (0, 3, 1). The line of solutions, which is represented as a bolded dotted line, passes through these points. This line passes through the values used to generate the data (1, 2, 2) and any other solution to the normal equations.† Typically, how "nature" generated the data would not be known to the researcher.

---

* If an error component were added to this simulation, it would not affect the X-matrix values. It would affect the distance of the line of solutions from the origin but not the fact that the solutions would be parallel to the null vector.
† Any two solutions to the normal equations can be used to determine the line of solutions.

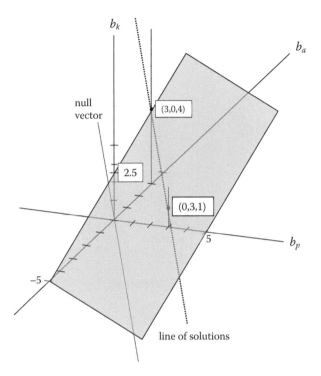

FIGURE 3.2
The geometry of linear dependency with linear coding of age, period, and cohort for the data in Equation (3.16).

The obstacle to finding a unique solution to this APC problem is that the line of solutions does not intersect the remaining plane at a single point; instead it lies on the remaining plane because the remaining equation is linearly dependent on the two equations used to form the line of solutions. For example, we can form the line of solution using the first two equations. Then the third equation is the remaining equation/plane. That plane is defined by the third normal equation as $-20b_a + 20b_p + 40b_k = 100$. The plane represented by this third equation must cross the age axis at -5.0, that is, at the point $(-5.0, 0.0, 0.0)$. When period and cohort are zero, the age coefficient must be -5.0 for the $X'y$ value to be 100. The plane must cross the period axis at 5.0, that is, at the point $(0.0, 5.0, 0.0)$, since when age is zero and cohort is zero, the period coefficient must be 5.0 for the $X'y$ value to be 100. The plane must cross the cohort axis at 2.5, that is, at the point $(0.0, 0.0, 2.5)$, since when age and period are zero, the cohort coefficient must then be 2.5 for the $X'y$ value to be 100.

Figure 3.2 depicts this plane crossing these points on the age, period, and cohort axes in the three-dimensional solution space for the APC model when age, period, and cohort are linearly coded. The line of solutions lies on this

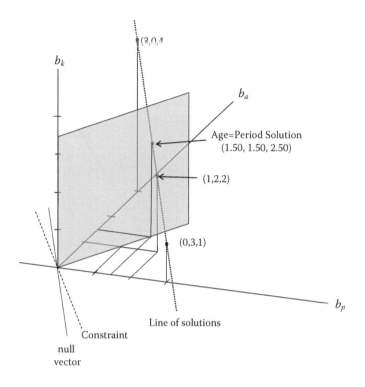

FIGURE 3.3
The geometry of the constrained solution for age1 = age2 with linear coding of age, period, and cohort for the data in Equation (3.16).

plane. The plane intersects the point $(3, 0, 4)$ and the point $(0, 3, 1)$, which are both on the line of solutions. This establishes that the line of solutions lies on the surface of this plane.

Figure 3.3 depicts the solution to Equation (3.16) when we constrain the age and period linear effects to be equal. Geometrically, two of the normal equations (again representing planes) are used to find their intersection, which is the line of solutions. The remaining plane is oriented so that it intersects the line of solutions at a unique point. In Figure 3.3, the constraint used is $(1, -1, 0)$, which means that $1b_a - 1b_p + 0b_k = 0$. This constrains the age coefficient and the period coefficient to be equal. The cohort coefficient can take on any value as far as the constraint is concerned, but its value will be determined by the constraint since the constraint will determine where the constrained plane intersects the line of solutions. The constraint is depicted in Figure 3.3 as the dashed line through the origin. It has a slope of −1 with respect to the age–period plane. The solution is constrained to be perpendicular (orthogonal) to this constraint. The same constraint holds at any value of b_k; for example, at 2 on the b_k dimension a unit increase in age is matched by a unit increase in period. This requires a plane that is perpendicular to

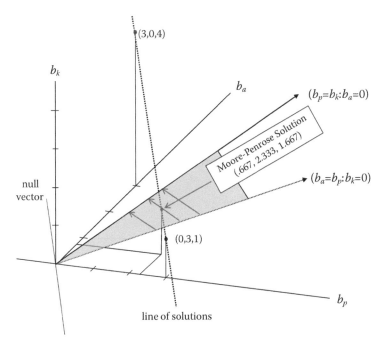

FIGURE 3.4
The geometry of the Moore–Penrose solution with linear coding of age, period, and cohort for the data in Equation (3.16).

the age–period plane with a slope of one on the age–period plane. This plane intersects the line of solutions at a unique point (1.50, 1.50, 2.50). All of the constrained solutions in constrained regression analysis are orthogonal to their constraint, that is, $(1.50, 1.50, 2.50)(1, -1, 0)' = 0$. Although this provides a unique solution, the substantive question is whether this particular solution provides good estimates of the parameters that generated the data.

Figure 3.4 depicts a more complicated constraint on the data, one that produces the Moore–Penrose solution. The Moore–Penrose solution is perpendicular to the null vector in the APC situation. In the case of linear coding of the APC model the null vector is $(1, -1, 1)'$ or in the three-space of the solutions to regression equations: $1 \times b_a - 1 \times b_p + 1 \times b_k = 0$. To conceptualize the direction of the constrained plane in this situation, note that when cohort equals zero we are on the age–period plane and that age and period must equal each other for the constraint to equal zero. We have depicted these equal values of the age and period coefficients with the dotted arrow in Figure 3.4 and note in parentheses $(b_a = b_p : b_k = 0)$: the age effect coefficient equals the period effect coefficient given that the cohort coefficient equals zero. The constrained plane must pass through this dotted line on the age–period plane. When the age coefficient is zero, we are on the period–cohort plane. For the constraint to hold, the period and cohort-coefficients must be equal, we use the solid arrow to depict these equal values of the period and cohort coefficients on the period–cohort plane ($b_p \cdot b_k \cdot b_a = 0$). The constrained plane lies on these lines. It is difficult to depict graphically, but the plane comes toward the reader from the bottom of the plane situated on the dotted line with an arrow tip and crossing through the solid line with an arrow tip. The plane, of course, extends beyond the triangular sliver depicted Figure 3.4. We have placed three arrows on this plane to give a sense of direction. Where this constrained plane intersects the line of solutions is the Moore–Penrose solution. It is a constrained solution. For our data the solution is (.667, 2.333, 1.667), which is orthogonal to its constraint (1, −1, 1), since (.667, 2.333, 1.667) (1, −1, 1)′ = 0.

3.5 Equivalence of the Geometric and Algebraic Solutions

These geometric solutions, of course, correspond to the algebraic solutions. Since $X'X$ is not of full column rank, it has no regular inverse and we cannot use the typical solution strategy of multiplying both sides of Equation (3.16) by $(X'X)^{-1}$ to obtain the unique solution vector: b. Geometrically, this is the linear dependency resulting from the line of solutions lying on the "remaining plane." Instead, as in Chapter 2, we must find a generalized inverse that will produce *a* least squares solution to the normal equations:

$$(X'X)^{-} X'Xb = (X'X)^{-} X'y. \tag{3.17}$$

As in Chapter 2, we can write this solution in a more explicit form as

$$b_{c1} = (X'X)^{-}_{c1} X'y, \tag{3.18}$$

where b_{c1} is a constrained solution to the normal equation under constraint $c1$, and $= (X'X)^{-}_{c1}$ is a generalized inverse based on this constraint. Geometrically, the generalized inverse constrains the direction of the remaining plane so that it intersects the line of solution at a point and thus provides *a* solution.

As in Chapter 2, the Mazumdar et al. (1980) procedure can be used to find a generalized inverse that will produce *a* solution under a particular constraint. We use their procedure to find a constrained solution for the data in Equation (3.16). For example, to impose the constraint $c1 = (1, -1, 0)$, which constrains the linear effect of age minus the linear effect of period plus zero times the linear effect of cohort to equal zero, we use Mazumdar et al.'s procedure. We replace the last row of $X'X$ in Equation (3.16) with (1, −1, 0), find the inverse of this new matrix, and then replace the final column of this matrix with zeros. This generalized inverse $(X'X)_{c1}^-$ times $X'y$ produces the solution to the normal equations under this constraint

$$(X'X)_{c1}^- \qquad X'y = b_{c1}$$

$$\begin{bmatrix} .025 & .025 & 0 \\ .025 & .025 & 0 \\ -.025 & .025 & 0 \end{bmatrix} \begin{bmatrix} -20 \\ 80 \\ 100 \end{bmatrix} = \begin{bmatrix} 1.5 \\ 1.5 \\ 2.5 \end{bmatrix}. \tag{3.19}$$

The solution is always orthogonal to its constraint, which we can verify for this data by calculating the dot product of the constraint vector $(1, -1, 0)$ and the solution vector: $(1.5, 1.5, 2.5)$. The result is zero indicating that the two vectors are orthogonal to each other. To find the solution orthogonal to the null vector (equivalent to the Moore–Penrose solution), we replace the last row of $X'X$ with $(1, -1, 1)$ and proceed with the Mazumdar et al. (1980) procedure. This constraint works because it is the null vector, and the Moore–Penrose solution produces the solution that is orthogonal to the null vector. The resulting solution is $(.667, 2.333, 1.667)$, and its dot product with the constraint is zero. The same results for the regression coefficients would be obtained if we used the raw data in Table 3.1 and included a vector of ones for the intercept. We worked without the intercept in this case so that we could stay in the three-dimensional situation and more easily conceptualize the solutions space geometrically.

If we had not centered these data on the means of each variable, the solution space would be four dimensional. There would be four normal equations and each one of them would be the equation for a three-dimensional hyperplane. Three of these hyperplanes would intersect in a line, but the remaining hyperplane would not intersect the line of solutions at a unique point. For constrained regression to work the direction of this remaining hyperplane would need to be constrained so that it intersects the line of solutions at a unique point. For example, if the order of the variables is intercept, age, period, and cohort, we would use the following constraint $(0, 1, -1, 0)$ to constrain the age and period coefficients to be equal. To obtain the Moore–Penrose solution, we would use $(0, 1, -1, 1)$ as the constraint.

3.6 Geometry of the Multiple Classification Model

The geometry of the multiple-classification model is more complex than the model based on linear coding, because it involves more dimensions: one for each of the parameters in the multiple-classification model. This geometry is illustrated using the 4 × 4 age–period matrix. In this situation X has 16 rows and 13 columns. The rows are for the 16 cell entries in the 4 × 4 age–period table, and the 13 columns represent the intercept, three age effects, three period effects, and six cohort effects (one age, one period, and one cohort category is used as a reference category). The $X'X$-matrix is 13 × 13 and the $X'y$-vector is 13 × 1 as is the b-vector. The APC problem persists in that the $X'X$-matrix is rank deficient by one.

The geometry is based on the 13 normal equations in $X'Xb = X'y$. Each row represents a 12-dimensional hyperplane. Any twelve of these hyperplanes intersect in a line: the line of solutions resides in the 13-dimensional solution space, but the remaining 12-dimensional hyperplane does not intersect the line of solutions at a unique point. The line of solutions lies on the remaining 12-dimensional hyperplane. (This occurs because of the linear dependency.) The remaining plane must be constrained in such a manner that it intersects the line of solutions. The hyperplane is rotated so that its direction is perpendicular to the constraint imposed by the researcher and, in general, it intersects the line of solutions at a point; the solution on the line of solutions is perpendicular to the constraint.[*]

Geometrically, we can view each of the solutions as lying on the line of solutions in 13-dimensional solution space. The line of solutions is represented by $(b_c^0 = b_{c1}^0 + sv)$. For example, the constraint for the age1 = age2 solution is $(0, 1, -1, 0, 0, \ldots, 0)$ and the remaining 12-dimensional hyperplane must be orthogonal to this constraint. In general, with a constraint, this hyperplane will intersect the line of solutions at a point. The line of solutions is parallel to the null vector.

For APC models of any dimension the extension to a model with m normal equations is straightforward. With m equations there are m-dimensions in the solution space. There are m equations representing m $(m-1)$-dimensional hyperplanes. The line of solutions (a line in m-space) is determined by the intersection of $m-1$ of these hyperplanes. Its vector equation is $b_c^0 = b_{c1}^0 + sv$, where b_c^0, b_{c1}^0, and v each have m-elements. The remaining hyperplane does not intersect the line of solutions. The single constraint that we place on the remaining hyperplane, in general, reorients it in the m-space and results in the constrained hyperplane intersecting the line of solutions at a single point that yields a solution to the system of m equations.

---

[*] Note the similarity to the case with three linearly coded and centered factors: age, period, and cohort previously discussed. There are three normal equations (rows) each of which represents a plane. Two of the planes intersect in a line, but the final plane does not intersect the line. This plane must be constrained to intersect with this line of solutions and it is perpendicular to its constraint. I used the term "in general" because one could constrain the remaining plane in such a way that it still did not intersect the line of solutions: that is, constrain it in such a way that it does not change its orientation.

3.7 Distance from Origin and Distance along the Line of Solutions

Figure 3.5 is designed as an aid to visualizing the relationships described in this section. It is a schematic representation, since there are likely to be many dimensions not shown in this figure. I have constructed a view of the plane that contains both the line of solution and the null vector. These both lie on a plane and we can imagine that plane as the surface of the page (this is possible because the null vector and the line of solutions are parallel to each other). The vector labeled w is a particular solution vector: the one that is perpendicular to the null vector (the intrinsic estimator [IE]/Moore–Penrose solution). The elements of a solution vector tell its position in the solution space. We know that it is a solution vector since its origin is $(0, 0, \ldots, 0)$ and its end point is on the line of solutions. The vector u is another constrained solution vector from the origin to the point on the line of solutions corresponding to that constrained solution. Both of these vectors are formed where the hyperplane cuts across the plane of this page.

We can calculate the length of a vector by squaring its elements, summing these squared elements, and taking the square root of this sum. For a vector labeled u in Figure 3.5 this is typically written as $\|u\|$; this is the dot product of the vector with itself square rooted: $\sqrt{u \cdot u}$. The length of the solution vectors w and u can be calculated, since the solution vector begins at the origin and ends at the line of solutions, it corresponds to the distance of the solution from the origin. We note that this distance is minimal for the solution that is orthogonal to the null vector w. This solution is a minimum norm solution.

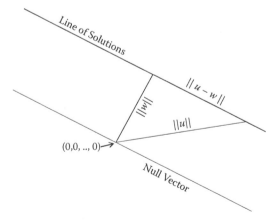

FIGURE 3.5
Schematic representation of the length of constrained solutions and the distance between solutions on the line of solutions.

The distance along the line of solutions between any two solutions can be calculated as the square root of the sum of the squared differences between the corresponding elements of two vectors: $\sqrt{(u-w)\cdot(u-w)}$. This is conventionally written as Distance = $\|u - w\|$. These are the formulas associated with finding the distance between two points. One other relationship is important. It is sv that determines the difference between two solution vectors on the line of solutions. It determines the element-by-element difference between two solutions. Therefore, it is not surprising that $|s|\|v\| = \|u - w\|$. That is, another way to calculate the distance between two solutions on the line of solutions is Distance = $|s|\|v\|$.

3.8 Empirical Example: Frost's Tuberculosis Data

I use data from the classic paper on tuberculosis by Frost (1939) discussed in Chapter 1. The data that appear in Table 1.2 of Chapter 1 are modified by combining the two age categories 0–4 and 5–9 into a single 10-year age category 0–9 (we averaged the rates per 100,000 in these two age groups) and we have eliminated the age category 70-plus. This leaves us with an age–period table in which each of the age groups is 10 years and the periods are separated by 10 years and the cohorts are 10-year cohorts (Table 3.2). The bottom left-hand entry of 402 is for the same cohort as the next entry on that minor diagonal of 115. It is for the same cohort, but when the cohort is 10–19.

The data are presented in rates per 100,000 people, and in our analyses these rates are logged. I usually log rates that are based on counts that are relatively rare since they are typically skewed to the right. It also makes the results closer to count model results. Four different constraints are used with this data; age1 = age2, cohort1 = cohort3, the Moore–Penrose constraint (the IE), and a zero linear trend (ZLT) for periods constraint.

TABLE 3.2

Age–Period-Specific Tuberculosis Mortality Rates (per 100,000) Based on Frost's (1939) Data

Age	1880	1890	1900	1910	1920	1930
60–69	475	340	304	246	172	95
50–59	366	325	267	252	171	127
40–49	364	336	253	253	175	118
30–39	378	368	296	253	164	115
20–29	444	361	288	207	149	81
10–19	126	115	90	63	49	21
0–9	402	314	170	115	66	26

Note: The bolded rates are for the cohort born from 1871 to 1880 that Frost labels as the 1880 cohort.

TABLE 3.3

Constrained Regression Results for the Logged Tuberculosis Rates for Males

Categories	age1 = age2	coh1 = coh3	IE	ZLT Period	Null Vector
Intercept	5.0900	5.0900	5.0900	5.0900	0
age 0–9	−2.6265	−0.3061	−0.0693	0.6900	−3
age 10–19	−2.6265	−1.0796	−0.9217	−0.4155	−2
age 20–29	−0.6794	0.0941	0.1730	0.4261	−1
age 30–39	0.2195	0.2195	0.2195	0.2195	0
age 40–49	1.0255	0.2521	0.1731	−0.0800	1
age 50–59	1.9092	0.3623	0.2044	−0.3018	2
age 60–69	2.7782	0.4578	0.2210	−0.5383	
period 1880	2.6846	0.7509	0.5536	−0.0791	2.5
period 1890	1.6889	0.5287	0.4103	0.0307	1.5
period 1900	0.5692	0.1825	0.1430	0.0165	0.5
period 1910	−0.4630	−0.0763	−0.0368	0.0898	−0.5
period 1920	−1.6142	−0.4540	−0.3356	0.0440	−1.5
period 1930	−2.8656	−0.9319	−0.7346	−0.1018	
cohort 1811–1820	−4.3895	−0.1355	0.2987	1.6907	−5.5
cohort 1821–1830	−3.7547	−0.2741	0.0811	1.2201	−4.5
cohort 1831–1840	−2.8426	−0.1355	0.1408	1.0267	−3.5
cohort 1841–1850	−1.9819	−0.0483	0.1491	0.7818	−2.5
cohort 1851–1860	−1.0709	0.0893	0.2077	0.5874	−1.5
cohort 1861–1870	−0.2537	0.1330	0.1725	0.2991	−0.5
cohort 1871–1880	0.6975	0.3107	0.2713	0.1447	0.5
cohort 1881–1890	1.4749	0.3147	0.1963	−0.1834	1.5
cohort 1891–1900	2.1885	0.2549	0.0576	−0.5752	2.5
cohort 1901–1910	2.8788	0.1717	−0.1046	−0.9905	3.5
cohort 1911–1920	3.3934	−0.0871	−0.4423	−1.5813	4.5
cohort 1921–1930	3.6601	−0.5939	−1.0280	−2.4201	

Note: The data are from Table 3.2.

Those results appear in Table 3.3. Note that the intercept is the same no matter what the constraint as are the coefficients for age group 30–39. This occurs because the null vector elements corresponding to these two coefficients are zero. No matter where on the line of solutions these solutions lie, these elements are the same, since for these elements the scalar times the null vector element is zero. The constrained solutions each produce solutions that are orthogonal to their constraints; this is easy to see with the first two constraints. The constraint for age is that age1 = age2; that is, (0 × int + 1 × age1 − 1 × age2 + 0 × age3, …, + 0 × coh11 = 0). It equals zero because the age 1 and age 2 estimates are the same. The solution in the coh1 = coh3 column is also orthogonal to its constraint, since all of the elements of that constraint are zero except those for cohort 1 and cohort 3 which are 1 and −1, respectively. To show that the IE solution is orthogonal to its constraint, we must find the dot product of this solution times the null vector. We have included the null vector for this 7×6 age–period table in the final column. The null vector has as many elements as there are independent variables in the X-matrix. That is, one for the intercept, one for each of the age categories except the reference category for age, one for each of the periods except for the reference category for periods, and one for each of the cohorts except for the reference category for cohorts: 23 (= 1 + 6 + 5 + 11). The solution space has 23 dimensions. The design matrix, the matrix of independent variables when postmultiplied by the null vector, results in a column vector of 23 zeros. The line of solutions is parallel to the null vector in this 23-dimensional solution space. The dot product of the IE solution vector (for the non-reference categories) and the null vector is zero; explicitly, $(0.00 \times 5.0900 - 3.0 \times -0.0693 - 2.0 \times -0.9217 \ldots 4.5 \times -0.4423 = 0.00)$. The IE solution is orthogonal to the null vector. The constraint for the zero linear trend for period is $(-5 \times \text{period}1880 - 4 \times \text{period}1890 - 3 \times \text{period}1900 - 2 \times \text{period}1910 - 1 \times \text{period}1920 = 0)$. That is, the dot product of $(0, 0, 0, 0, 0, 0, 0, -5, -4, -3, -2, -1, 0, \ldots, 0)$ times the solution for the zero linear trend in the periods vector (not including the reference categories) is zero. These vectors are orthogonal to their constraints (perpendicular in the 23-dimensional solution space).

The vector equation for a line $b_c^0 = b_{c1}^0 + sv$ describes the relationship of the best fitting solutions to one another. In terms of the line of solutions, the distance that two solutions b_{c1}^0 and b_{c2}^0 are apart is $|s| \, \|v\|$. Taking one of these constrained solutions (the one based on the age1 = age2 constraint), we can show that the other solutions can be generated by selecting the appropriate value of the scalar s. Given our choice for the "reference" constrained solution of $b_{age1=age2}$, $s = -0.773$, for obtaining the solution under the cohort constraint; $s = -0.852$, for obtaining the solution under the intrinsic estimator constraint; and $s = -1.105$, for obtaining the solution under the zero linear trend for periods constraint. These solutions lie on a single line, since they are all derivable using the vector equation for a line: $b_c^0 = b_{c1}^0 + sv$. We can calculate the distance of each of these solutions from the age1 = age2 solution using either the formula $|s| \, \|v\|$ and substituting the values of s derived earlier or $\|u - w\|$ where u is the age1 = age2 solution vector and w is the other solution vector. The formulas provide the same results for the distance between solutions on the line of solutions: age1 = age2 to coh1 = coh3 is 9.249, age1 = age2 to IE is 10.193, age1 = age2 to zero linear trend period is 13.220.

We can calculate the distance of each of these solutions on the line of solutions from the origin by squaring the elements of the solution vector, summing these squared elements, and taking the square root of this sum. The lengths of these solution vectors are $\|b_{age1=age2}^0\| = 11.487$, $\|b_{coh1=coh3}^0\| = 5.380$, $\|b_{ie}^0\| = 5.297$, and $\|b_{ZLTperiod}^0\| = 6.101$. As geometrically required, the distance of the intrinsic estimator solution from the origin is shortest. This must be the case because it is the solution on the line of solutions that is orthogonal to the null vector making it orthogonal to the line of solutions.

This geometry helps us understand two properties of the solution that is perpendicular to the null vector. (1) There is *a sense in which this solution is an average of all of the possible constrained solutions* to the just identified multiple-classification APC model. The idea behind this "sense" is that if we conceive of an infinite number of solutions spread out across the line of solutions (or, if you like, at distances from each other of .01), there is a sense in which the middle of that distribution of solutions is at the point perpendicular to the null vector. In this sense, this solution is at the "balance point" in the center of this line of solutions. This is probably the reason for the following two statements from the literature. Smith (2004:116) states: "There is also a sense in which the IE [intrinsic estimator] is an average of Constrained Generalized Linear Model (CGLIM) estimates." Press, Teukolsky, Vetterling, and Flannery (1992:62) note that in the rank deficient by one situation, "If we want to single out one particular member of the solution-set of vectors as representative, we might want to pick the one with the smallest length." In their statement Press et al. mention the second property. (2) The solution perpendicular to the null vector *is a minimum norm solution* (shortest distance from the origin to the solution). This can be considered a statistical property of this solution. For example, in the least squares situation we select the solution vector b that minimizes the distance: $\|y - Xb\|$. In the rank deficient by one case, which we encounter in the APC model, this criterion of best fit does not yield a unique solution because any solution on the line of solutions minimizes this distance. Only one solution, however, minimizes $\|y-Xb\|$ and $\|b\|$, that is, the perpendicular solution. This property is related to the fact that the variance of the perpendicular solution is less than that for the other constrained solutions.

3.9 Summarizing Some Important Features from the Geometry of APC Models

The quotation at the beginning of this chapter emphasizes the importance of combining a geometric and algebraic view of, in our case, the APC model. With both views in hand our understanding of the problems and solutions is enhanced. Understanding the geometry makes us less likely to lose our intuitive sense of the problem in the complexity of algebraic manipulations. Understanding the geometry will prevent us from being misled by complex geometric arguments. I illustrate this point with a simple illustration of the perpendicular solution at the end of this chapter.

3.9.1 Solutions Lie on a Line in Multidimensional Space

That the solutions lie on a line in multidimensional space not only indicates that there are an infinite number of solutions to the APC model, all of which are equally good in terms of fit, but also eliminates an infinite number of other solutions that do not lie on the line of solutions. This fact is used in Chapter 4 to derive a number of "estimable functions." These functions (for example) uniquely estimate the second differences of age coefficients, period coefficients, and cohort coefficients; they estimate the deviations of age coefficients from the linear trend in age coefficients, the deviations of period coefficients from the linear trend in period coefficients, and the deviations of cohort coefficients from the linear trend in cohort coefficients; and they uniquely estimate the predicted values of the outcome variable y. These solutions are unique in the sense that they are the same for any of the constrained solutions and, importantly, are the same as those for the parameters that generated the outcome data.

With algebraic approaches it is easy to overlook the line of solutions and simply note that the regression coefficients are not identified, that the matrix of independent variables is not invertible, that a linear dependency exists, and that there are an infinite number of solutions. But the geometry emphasizes that we know much more than that. We know the combinations of regression coefficients that satisfy the best fit criterion. We also have an intuitive (geometrical) grasp of what it means for the dot product of two vectors to be zero.

3.9.2 Distances as Geometric Insights

The geometric approach provides a concrete understanding of the minimum norm solution. The distance of any constrained solution on a line of solutions from the origin of the multidimensional solution space is $\|b_{c1}^0\|$. The solution vector with the shortest distance (length) is the minimum norm solution. The geometry of the situation makes it clear that the minimum norm solution is the solution that is perpendicular to the null vector (that is, the IE/Moore–Penrose solution). The geometric approach also provides a concrete understanding of the relationship of the solutions on the line of solutions in terms of their distance from each other on the line of solutions. Since sv is added to one solution to get to another solution, the geometrical approach shows that they are separated by a distance of $|s|\,\|v\|$.

3.9.3 Understanding How Constrained Regression Solves the Rank Deficient Case

From the geometric perspective the problem with rank deficiency in the APC model is that, even though we can determine the line of solutions by the intersection of $m-1$ of the hyperplanes that represent $m-1$ of the normal equations, there is always a hyperplane left over that does not intersect the line of solutions. Statistically, any of the solutions on the line of solutions might represent the parameters that generated the outcome variable. Some of them, however, might be rejected on the basis of what is known about tuberculosis. For example, we would not constrain the cohort effect to increase over time given what we know about exposure to tuberculosis and its typical latency period over time. In the same sense a criminologist would be unlikely to choose a constraint with a positive trend for age to identify an age–period–cohort model of homicide offending in the United States. The important point is that any solution on the line is a potential solution and, if we do not bring some "outside information" to bear, perhaps an equally likely solution. What constrained regression does is to change the direction of the remaining hyperplane so that it is orthogonal to the constraint, and the hyperplane intersects the line of solutions at a single point. This provides an unbiased solution to the APC problem *under the constraint*.

3.10 Problem with Mechanical Constraints

When using constrained regression to solve the APC problem, how good a solution is depends mainly on the constraint used to obtain it. If the constraint matches the way in which nature generated the data, then the entire solution will be consistent with the way the data were generated (always with the caveat that the full APC specification is the correct specification). The term "mechanical constraint" means that the approach generally applies the same constraint or procedure to all data sets. Mechanical constraints will provide an unbiased solution for parameters associated with how the data were generated, only if the constraint is consistent with the way nature generated the outcome values.

It may be the case that a particular mechanical solution is more efficient in terms of the standard errors being smaller than other constrained solutions, or that the distance from the origin to the solution is smaller with a particular estimate, or that the solution is orthogonal to the null vector (Yang, Fu, and Land 2004; Yang, Schulhofer-Wohl, Fu, and Land 2008), or that it is a maximum entropy solution (Browning, Crawford, and Knoef 2012), or that it is the solution provided by a principal component regression analysis (Fu 2000; Kupper, Janis, Salama, Yoshizawa, Greenberg 1983). These approaches use no information about the substantive content of the data or problem in order to identify the APC model. For example, in the rank deficient by one situation, which occurs with APC models, the intrinsic estimator uses a constraint equivalent to that imposed by the Moore–Penrose solution as the constraint for finding the solution to the APC problem. Yang et al. (2008) note several potential statistical advantages of this estimator: minimum variances for the parameters, the shortest length of the solution vector from the origin to the line of solution of any constrained solution, the solution being perpendicular to the null vector, and they suggest that (2008:1697) "the IE holds the potential for applications not only to APC analysis but also to similar problems of structural underidentification in sociology."

The *logic* of this sort of method is perhaps easiest to see in the situation in which there are just two independent variables. Imagine that a researcher wants to measure the effects of age on support for same-sex marriage. She collects data from subjects who are 21 to 60 years of age in a single survey conducted 2013, and she linearly codes the data. The researcher is sophisticated enough to recognize that this phenomenon could be related to age, but that each of the ages also represents a different cohort. That is, she has two independent variables to explain the age distribution of favorability to same-sex marriage: age and cohort. She knows that the model is underidentified, since Period – Age = Cohort and in this cross-sectional study period is fixed. She decides to use constrained regression so that she can estimate the effects of both age and cohort on support of same-sex marriage.

There is a problem, because the results for the coefficients for age and cohort will differ depending on the constraint chosen by the researcher. She knows, however, that she can use the Moore–Penrose generalized inverse and that the resulting solution will have some nice statistical properties: minimum norm solution, smallest variance, and being orthogonal to the null vector. She does not attempt to justify this constraint substantively, because there is a literature that supports using the Moore–Penrose inverse in such situations. Centered data are used so that the logic of her analysis can be seen geometrically in a two-dimensional solutions space.

Figure 3.6 is based on the following example data for the normal equations that might be calculated from the age, cohort, and support for same-sex marriage data collected by the investigator:

$$
\begin{matrix} X'X & \qquad\qquad b - X'y \end{matrix}
$$

$$
\begin{bmatrix} 1050 & -1050 \\ -1050 & 1050 \end{bmatrix} \begin{bmatrix} b_a \\ b_k \end{bmatrix} = \begin{bmatrix} -2100 \\ 2100 \end{bmatrix}. \tag{3.19}
$$

It is not surprising that the $X'X$ matrix indicates a linear dependency between the independent variables: the first column is equal to minus one times the second column, and the second row is equal to the minus one times the first row. $X'X$ must have this symmetrical form, since age and cohort are perfectly negatively correlated and have the same variance. The two entries in $X'y$ must also be the same but of opposite sign. Since age is in the first row of X' and is multiplied by the column y, we expect this dot product to be negative: we expect age to be negatively related to support for same-sex marriage. The linear dependency makes the signs of the $X'y$ opposite for the age and cohort rows and of the same absolute value (remember the variables have been centered for this analysis). Each of the normal equations represents the equation for a line. Figure 3.6 depicts this relationship. Because of the linear

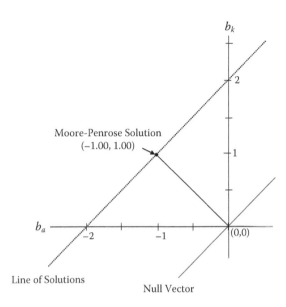

FIGURE 3.6
Moore–Penrose solution for a rank deficient by one problem in two-dimensional solution space.

dependency, the two lines will coincide with each other: one line lies on the other line. They do not intersect at a unique point to provide a unique solution. We establish the line of solutions by noting that when the cohort effect is zero, b_a must equal –2. That is, the line crosses the age axis at –2, (–2, 0), and when age is zero for the normal equation to provide a correct solution, b_k must be 2. The line of solutions crosses the cohort axis at 2, (0, 2). The null vector (which is unique up to multiplication by a scalar) is (1, 1). It must pass through the origin (0, 0), and note in Figure 3.6 that it is parallel to the line of solutions.

As depicted in Figure 3.6, the solution generated by the Moore–Penrose generalized inverse is orthogonal to the null vector: (–1.00, 1.00)(1, 1)′ = 0. It has the shortest distance of any solution vector from the origin to the line of solutions. Associated with this, it has the minimum variance property. The researcher does not have to use theory or substantive knowledge to set this "mechanical constraint." We can also obtain this solution by using principle component regression. It is also the maximum entropy solution.

The following question, however, must be asked: Even though this solution based on the Moore–Penrose generalized inverse has these properties, should we feel reasonably confident that the effect of age on support for same-sex marriage is of the same magnitude as the effect of cohort on support for same-sex marriage, but of opposite sign? The question for the researcher in this substantive area is whether this mechanical solution produces an adequate solution to the substantive question. Does it answer the question about the relative importance of age and the relative importance of cohort to support for same-sex marriage in this context? Since any point on the line of solutions produces the same output values (**predicted values**) for support for same-sex marriage, the model fit cannot adjudicate between the different solutions. In its starkest form, the Moore–Penrose constraint can produce an answer to the following equation: $x + y = 10$. The answer is that both x and y equal 5. Despite the fact that this answer has some nice statistical properties, how much confidence should we have (if this were a substantive problem) that this answer is correct in terms of how nature produced this outcome value?

A recommendation sometimes made in the APC context is that if adding one of the factors (age, period, or cohort) to a model does not significantly increase the fit of the model, then one should use the model without that factor. This example clearly demonstrates the problem with such a strategy. Since age and cohort are linearly dependent and they are linearly coded, they explain the same amount of variance singly that they could explain in a model in which both of them appear. That is, adding one of them to a model that contains the other does not improve the fit of the model. If we leave cohort out of the model and run a bivariate regression with age as the independent variable, the coefficient for age is –2; if we leave age out of the model and regress support for same-sex marriage on cohort, the coefficient for cohort is 2. The problem with such a strategy is that without the left out factor in the model, the other factor or factors take credit for any linear effect it might have, and that effect can be substantial. I expand on this theme in later chapters.

3.11 Discussion

There is a sense in which people are visual creatures even when reasoning: "I'll believe it when I see it," "Oh, I see how that works." Understanding the geometry of APC models allows us to see what the algebra is doing and provides added insights. Visualizing the infinite number of solutions that do not solve the APC model and the infinite number of solutions that do solve the APC model provides a deeper understanding of the identification problem. We can also see how this underidentification is "remedied" using a constrained estimator (changing the direction of the remaining hyperplane so that it intersects the line at a unique point). It provides a stronger sense of what it means to say that a solution is perpendicular to its constraint (not only is the dot product zero, but it really is geometrically perpendicular).

The geometrical view provides us with another sense of what sv means, the term that links all of the constrained solutions on the line of solutions. It determines the distance between solutions on the line of solutions, which is $|s| \, \|v\|$. The geometrical view allows us to concretely see the distance of a solution vector from the origin to the solution line and visualize the relation-ships of solutions to one another. It provides a rationale for the argument that the perpendicular solution might be the "most representative" solution. It strengthens our understanding of constrained estimators and provides another tool for evaluating and comparing constrained estimates.

In the next chapter, the fact that all of the "best fitting" solutions lie on a line in multidimensional space is used to derive a series of estimable functions. These functions are the same for all of the constrained solutions and there-fore for the parameters that generated the outcome data. These include such valuable functions as the deviations of age, period, and cohort effects from the linear trends for the age effects, period effects, and cohort effects, and the second differences for age effects, for period effects, and for cohort effects. There are several other estimable functions that can be derived from the line of solutions and a method for doing so is presented in detail.

Appendix 3.1

This chapter deals with m independent variables and m normal equations (for ease of presentation, I assumed that the variables were in deviation score form). But if the data is in raw score form and a column of ones is added to the X-matrix, this is just another parameter estimate and it adds another dimension to the solution space. For example, if there are three independent variables, then there are four columns in the X-matrix and $X'Xb = X'y$ is a set of four normal equations.

I present five points that should be helpful in thinking about the "behavior" of hyperplanes in the m-space. In the case of normal equations:

1. There are m equations (hyperplanes) and an m-dimensional solu-tion space.

2. Each of the normal equations is an $(m - 1)$-dimensional hyperplane.

3. When hyperplanes representing two linearly independent $(m - 1)$-dimensional hyperplanes intersect their intersection produces an $(m - 2)$-dimensional hyperplane. (Think of a three-dimensional space where each of the normal equations represents a plane [a $(3 - 1)$-dimensional hyperplane] and the intersection of these two planes is a line [a $(3 - 2)$-dimensional hyperplane]).

4. The intersection of an $(m - p)$-dimensional hyperplane with an $(m - 1)$-dimensional hyperplane is an $(m - (p + 1))$-dimensional hyperplane. Thus, in the case of three centered independent vari-ables and no linear dependency, the first two planes intersect in a $(3 - 2)$-dimensional hyperplane and this hyperplane intersects

with the remaining hyperplane in a point. The intersection is a $(3 - (2 + 1))$-dimensional hyperplane or a zero-dimensional hyperplane, which is a point.

5. With traditional APC models $m - 1$ of the equations are linearly independent. Thus, $m - 1$ of the $(m - 1)$-dimensional hyperplanes intersect to produce an $m - (m - 1)$-dimensional hyperplane. That is, a one-dimensional hyperplane: the line of solutions. The final hyperplane does not intersect this line of solutions in a point, since the line of solutions lies on the remaining $(m - 1)$-dimensional hyperplane. This is why it is necessary to constrain the direction of this hyperplane in order for it to intersect the line of solutions at a point.

References

Blalock, H. M. Jr. 1967. Status inconsistency, social mobility, status integration and structural effects. *American Sociological Review* 32:790–801.

Box, J.F. 1978. *R.A. Fisher, the Life of a Scientist*. New York: Wiley.

Browning, M., I. Crawford, and M. Knoef. 2012. The age period cohort problem: Set identification and point identification. http://www.economics.ox.ac.uk/members/ian.crawford/papers/apc.pdf

Cohen, J., P. Cohen, S.G. West, and L.S. Aiken. 2003. *Applied Multiple Regression/Correlation Analysis in the Behavioral Sciences* (3rd edition). Mahwah, NJ: Erlbaum.

Duncan, O.D. 1966. Methodological issues in the analysis of social mobility. In *Social Structure and Mobility in Economic Development*, eds. N.J. Smelser and S.M. Lipset, 51–97. Chicago: Aldine.

Fox, J. 2008. *Applied Regression Analysis and Generalized Linear Models* (2nd edition). Thousand Oaks, CA: Sage.

Frost, W.H. 1939. The age selection of mortality from tuberculosis in successive decades. *American Journal of Hygiene* 30:91–96. Reprinted in the *American Journal of Epidemiology*, 1995, 141–9.

Fu, W.J. 2000. Ridge estimator in singular design with applications to age-period-cohort analysis of disease rates. *Communications in Statistics–Theory and Method* 29:263–78.

Kendall, M.G. 1961. *A Course in the Geometry of n Dimensions*. London: Charles Griffin & Company.

Kupper, L.L., J.M. Janis, I.A. Salama, C.N. Yoshizawa, and B.G. Greenberg. 1983. Age-period-cohort analysis: An illustration of the problems in assessing interaction in one observation per cell data. *Communications in Statistics* 12:2779–807.

Mazumdar, S., C.C. Li, and G.R. Bryce. 1980. Correspondence between a linear restriction and a generalized inverse in linear model analysis. *The American Statistician* 34:103–5.

O'Brien, R.M. 2012. Visualizing rank deficient models: A row equation geometry of rank deficient matrices and constrained regression. *PLoS ONE* 7(6):e38923 doi: 10.1371/journal.pone.0038923.

Press, W.H., S.A. Teukolsky, W.T. Vetterling, and B.P. Flannery. 1992. *Numerical Recipes in C: The Art of Scientific Computing*. New York: Cambridge University Press.

Rodgers, W.L. 1982. Estimable functions of age, period, and cohort effects. *American Sociological Review* 47:774–87.

Smith, H.L. 2004. Response: Cohort analysis redux. *Sociological Methodology* 34: 111–9.

Strang, G. 1998. *Introduction to Linear Algebra* (2nd edition). Wellesley, MA: Wellesley-Cambridge Press.

Yang, Y., W.J. Fu, and K.C. Land. 2004. A methodological comparison of age-period-cohort models: Intrinsic estimator and conventional generalized linear models. In *Sociological Methodology*, ed. R.M. Stolzenberg, 75–110. Oxford: Basil Blackwell.

Yang, Y., S. Schulhofer-Wohl, W.J. Fu, and K.C. Land. 2008. The intrinsic estimator for age-period-cohort analysis: What it is and how to use it. *American Journal of Sociology* 113:1697–736.

4

*Estimable Functions Approach**

For now we see through a glass darkly...

I Corinthians 13:12

4.1 Introduction

This first part of the opening biblical quote is particularly appropriate for this chapter. From the previous chapters it is clear that it is not possible, in some mechanical manner, to obtain unbiased estimates of the age, period, and cohort parameters that generated the outcome values, even though these generating parameters are of central interest in the substantive fields that use age–period–cohort (APC) models.[†] For the individual age, period, and cohort coefficients there are an infinite number of estimates that fit the data equally well; therefore, we cannot use the likelihood of the estimated coefficients based on the data to determine the most likely generating parameters. Despite this limitation, I examine and extend a method that provides a partial view of the relationships between ages, periods, and cohorts to the outcome values. These estimates are unbiased estimates for the linear combination of the underlying data generating parameters.

This partial view includes, for example, the following *estimable functions*: Second differences – Difference of differences: [(age3 – age2) – (age2 – age1)]; the deviations of the period coefficients from linear trends in the period coefficients; and the least squares and generalized linear models predicted values of the outcome variable. These estimable functions are identified. They provide unique estimates that do not depend on the constraint used. The literature on estimable functions in APC analysis is vast (for example, Clayton

---

[*] Parts of this chapter are based on O'Brien (2014).

[†] As with any regression model the ability to obtain an unbiased estimate of the generating parameters depends upon the model being correctly specified. In this chapter the assumption is made that the full set of age, period, and cohort effects is the correct specification. One can obtain an unbiased estimate of these effects using constrained regression only if the constraint is true for the generating parameters. In constrained regression, correctly specifying this constraint is an additional assumption that must be met for the full APC model to be correctly specified. Correctly specifying this constraint is not required for unbiased estimates of estimable functions.

and Schifflers 1987; Holford 1983, 1985, 1991, 2005; Kupper, Janis, Karmous, and Greenberg 1985; O'Brien 2014; O'Brien and Stockard 2009; Robertson, Gandini, and Boyle 1999; Rodgers 1982; Tarone and Chu 1996).

This chapter shows how estimable functions work in the APC context and provides a unified approach to the derivation of such functions. To accomplish this, I use some important relationships derived in earlier chapters (null vectors, the line of solutions, generating parameters, and constrained solutions). The primary relationship relied on is that the best fitting solutions to the just identified APC model all lie on a single line in multidimensional space $(b_c^0 = b_{c1}^0 + sv)$. Estimable functions are linear combinations of the solutions on this line, and these linear combinations are invariant to the constraint used to solve the equations. They are, therefore, unbiased estimates of the same linear combination of the unknown parameters that generated the outcome data, since estimates of these parameters lie on this line of solutions.

When using the line of solutions to derive estimable functions, the null vector plays a major role, so I briefly review the patterning of the null vector. The null vector elements are ordered so that the element corresponding to the intercept appears first, then those for the age coefficients, the period coefficients, and the cohort coefficients. These groups of coefficients are separated by a semicolon for clarity. The null vector for the effect coded variables for a 5×5 age–period table is $v = (0; -2, -1, 0, 1; 2, 1, 0, -1; -4, -3, -2, -1, 0, 1, 2, 3).^*$

Note the interesting form of the null vector: the coding for the age group null vector elements consists of a linear trend increasing from the youngest to oldest age group, an opposite trend is associated with the coding of the period elements, and the trend for the cohort elements is in the same direction as that for age groups. Since the null vector is unique only up to multiplication by a scalar, we can shift the direction of these trends by multiplying the null vector by a negative number. In either case the trend for the age and cohort elements are in the same direction and the trend of the period elements is in the opposite direction. These fundamental relationships play a role in the derivation of several important estimable functions. I begin with the classic definition of an estimable function.

4.2 Estimable Functions

Searle (1971:180) provides a classic exposition of estimable functions. He defines an estimable function as "[b]asically ... a linear function of the parameters [β, the generating parameters] for which an estimator can be found from b^0 [our b_c^0] that is invariant to whatever solution of the normal

---

* There are no null vector elements for the reference groups (here the oldest age group, the most recent period, and the most recent cohort).

equations is for b^0." That is, for the APC situation, a linear combination of the parameters that generated the outcome values for which an (unbiased) estimate can be found from the same linear combination of any one of the constrained solutions. Searle (1971:162) makes a very strong assessment of the value of estimable functions: "They all have the property that they are invariant to whatever solution is obtained to the normal equations. Because of this invariance property they are the only functions that can be of interest, so far as estimation of the parameters of a linear model is concerned."[*]
I would likely not conclude that they are the only functions that can be of interest, but Searle's position is not without merit. Searle (p. 185) provides a necessary and sufficient condition for a linear combination of these solutions, $q'b_c^0$, to be an estimable function. He defines H as equal to $GX'X$, where G is a just identified generalized inverse; the requirement for $q'b_c^0$ to be an estimable function is that $q'H = q'$.

As an example, we later show that some second differences (differences between differences) are estimable [e.g., (age3 − age2) − (age2 − age1)]. In this case, if the order of the columns in X is intercept, age groups, periods, and cohorts then $q' = (0, +1, -2, +1, 0, 0, ..., 0)$. For $q'b_c^0$ (the second difference of these age coefficients in the solution vector) to be an estimable function, the necessary and sufficient condition is that $q'GX'X = q'$. Note that q' is a vector that when applied to the solution vector produces a simple linear combination of the elements in the solution vector: the potential estimable function. G is a just identifying generalized inverse. Although Searle's derivation uses ordinary least squares, his approach and the approach used in this text are equally valid for ordinary least squares (OLS) and generalized linear models.[†]

There are some less formal ways to recognize estimable functions by their characteristics. Holford (1985:833) states: "These functions are not affected by arbitrary choices that a data analyst might make by setting up constraints, but are the same for all constraints." That these linear combinations are the same for the generating parameters is what makes them useful, they tell us some things about how "nature generated the outcome data" in terms of the APC specification.

---

[*] The term *estimable* is sometimes used to mean that one can obtain unbiased estimates under a constraint. Mason, Mason, Winsborough, and Poole (1973:248) state, "age, cohort and period effects are estimable under the assumption that two coefficients are equal within one of the three dimensions." This is different from the estimable functions discussed in this chapter that are the same no matter which constraint is used. The estimable coefficients in a constrained regression are not all the same across whatever constraint is used.

[†] Although constrained estimators provide the individual age, period, and cohort effects as estimable functions *under the constraint*, these estimates vary using different constraints, and the full set of individual coefficients will not meet Searle's (1971) criterion for estimability. For example, using a constrained estimate for the 5 × 5 age–period table and $q = (0, 1, 0, ... , 0)$ for checking age 1 for estimability, we find that the criterion is not met: $q'H \ne q'$. The age 1 effect is not estimable. When $q = (0, 0, 0, 1, 0, ... 0)$, then $q'H = q'$ showing that the age 3 effect is estimable for the 5 × 5 age–period table. We will discuss the estimability of such individual coefficients later in this chapter.

In the published APC literature, the methods for demonstrating that a particular function is estimable cover a range of approaches from simple algebra analogous to that used in path analysis (Jagodzinski 1984) to proofs based on matrix algebra (Holford 1983), with a potpourri of other methods (Clayton and Schifflers 1987; Rodgers 1982; Tarone and Chu 1996). This chapter presents a method that can derive the estimable functions that appear in the literature and can be utilized to derive new ones (O'Brien 2012a). The approach can be used with different coding for the X-matrix (for example, effect coding or dummy variable coding), but the method will be demonstrated with effect coding.

4.3 $l'sv$ Approach for Establishing Estimable Functions in Age–Period–Cohort (APC) Models

The key to this approach is that any of the least squares and generalized linear model solutions, in the rank deficient by one case, lie on a line in m-dimensional solution space. The vector equation for this line is $b_c^0 = b_{c1}^0 + sv$. In a very real sense, *this is what we know about the solutions to the APC model that contains all of the age, period, and cohort coefficients.*

The estimable functions are particular linear combinations of the solutions that lie on this line. Not all linear combinations are estimable functions, but one characteristic of the ones that are is that they are invariant across the constrained solutions, and they are true not only for all of the constrained solutions but also for the generating parameters, which lie on this line. The $l'sv$ approach depends on the fact that the solutions that lie on the line of solutions $b_c^0 = b_{c1}^0 + sv$ differ from one another by sv. More formally, taking a linear combination (l) of both sides of $b_c^0 = b_{c1}^0 + sv$ yields ($l'b_c^0 = l'b_{c1}^0 + l'sv$). This is a set of three dot products, and the question is whether the linear combination of the solutions $l'b_c^0$ and $l'b_{c1}^0$ are equal for all values of s. This will be the case, if and only if the linear combination $l'sv = 0$ for all values of s. If this criterion is met, then the linear combination must be the same across all of the constrained solutions on the line of solutions. When we apply this criterion, sometimes we will take advantage of the fact that since s is a scalar if $l'v = 0$, $l'sv = 0$ for all values of s.

In terms of precedence, this criterion was suggested by Kupper et al. (1985) in an appendix to their article (Appendix B). Their derivation of $b_c^0 = b_{c1}^0 + sv$ is quite different from the one presented in Chapter 2, and they provide only one example in which the linear combination is not estimable and note that orthogonal polynomial coefficients for quadratic and higher order effects can be shown to be estimable functions using this criterion. Their approach drew the following unenthusiastic comment from Holford (1985:833): "There are several ways of showing estimability, and this has been discussed by Rodgers (1982) and Holford (1983). In their Appendix B, Kupper et al. (1985) also present a way of testing for estimability; however, their claim for greater simplicity is debatable."

In this chapter, the $l'sv$ approach is embraced and extended. I view this approach as a key to unifying the growing number of known estimable functions for APC models that have been derived by many authors. When using this approach, one must be careful to follow the criterion $l'sv = 0$ quite carefully. It is a particular linear combination of coefficients that is estimable; and if this particular linear combination is not meaningful or helpful, it is of little use. For example, using our ordering of the intercept, age, period, and cohort coefficients, we can show in the 5 × 5 age–period table that the age1 coefficient is not estimable. The dot product of $l' = (0, 1, 0, 0, ..., 0)$ times the null vector $(0,-2,-1, 0, 1, 2, 1, ..., 3)'$ is –2, so the age1 coefficient is not estimable. Another meaningful and potentially helpful function is the second difference of the age coefficients: (age3 – age2) – (age2 – age1) or (age1 –2 × age2 + age3). In this case, the appropriate linear combination to check for estimability is the dot product of $(0, 1,-2, 1, 0, 0, ..., 0) × (0,-2,-1, 0, 1, 2, ..., 3)'$ which is zero. This second difference is an estimable function. It is the same for all constrained solutions and for the parameters that generated the outcome data.

On the other hand, there are estimable functions that may not be particularly meaningful or helpful. For example, in the 5 × 5 age–period matrix the age1 plus period 1 effect is estimable. Here, $l' = (0, 1, 0, 0, 0, 1, 0, ..., 0)$, which when multiplied times the null vector equals zero (it also meets Searle's criterion). It is the same for all constrained solutions, but this particular estimable function is not likely to be very helpful for researcher in most situations.

In this context, we address the intrinsic estimator (IE) as an estimable function. Yang and associates (2004, 2008, 2013) state that the IE is an estimable function using the criteria suggested by Kupper et al. (1985). They use $l' = (I - \beta_0 \beta_0')$, where β_0 is the normed null vector, and show that $l'v = 0$, where 0 is a vector of zeros. Note that $(I - \beta_0 \beta_0')$ is a matrix not a vector as specified by Kupper et al., and 0 is a vector of zeros. Still one can test whether each of the rows of $(I - \beta_0 \beta_0')$ are estimable functions by multiplying each of its rows by the null vector. We find that each row of $(I - \beta_0 \beta_0')$ times the null vector equals zero. *Each of these rows is a linear combination of the IE solution vector that is estimable.* This would essentially solve the APC identification problem, if the linear combinations produced by each of these rows estimated a different age, period, and cohort coefficient, but they do not. In fact, most of the estimable functions produced by these rows are not very helpful linear combinations. Using the 5 × 5 age–period matrix and constructing $(I - \beta_0 \beta_0')$, we find that the first row of $(I - \beta_0 \beta_0')$ produces a meaningful linear combination when postmultiplied by the null vector, since it is a 1 followed by all zeros and establishes that that the intercept is optimable (as it is for all constrained estimators that use effect coding). The second row, however, is (0.000, 0.929, −0.036, 0.000, 0.036, 0.071, 0.036, 0.000, −0.036, −0.143, −0.107, −0.071,−0.036, 0.000, 0.036, 0.071, 0.107), that is, 0 times the intercept plus 0.929 times the age1 effect minus 0.036 times the age2 effect, and so on. This linear combination of these age, period, and cohort effects will be the same no matter which constrained estimator is used. The crucial question is whether this linear combination of the effect estimates is meaningful as an estimate of the age 1 effect. The entire $(I - \beta_0 \beta_0')$ matrix is reproduced as Table A4.1.1 in Appendix 4.1. Most of the estimable functions derived from the rows of this table are not likely to be very meaningful or helpful linear combinations. When we interpret the coefficients from the IE, we must remember that coefficients such as the age1 coefficient are not estimable functions for age1, but rather for some other linear combination of effect coefficients. Kupper et al. (1985) using their criterion demonstrated that $(0, 1, 0, 0, \ldots, 0)$ is not an estimable function (Searle's criterion produces the same result). In fact, the age1 coefficient from the IE is not an estimable function for age1, but represents a quite different estimable function as shown above.[*] The individual age, period, and cohort coefficients are not estimable, except in certain special cases and then only certain of the coefficients are estimable (as will be shown shortly).

In my judgment, it is confusing to label a solution vector such as the IE as an estimable function when the individual elements of that vector are not all estimable functions that correspond to the elements of that solution vector. It is typical to say that a linear combination is an estimable function of that linear combination of the solution vector; for example, the second differences are estimable, the age1 coefficient is not estimable. Yang and associates (2004, 2008, 2013) instead test a set of linear combinations and find that each of these linear combinations is an estimable function. Then they label the IE solution vector as an estimable function. The problem is that a researcher might take this to mean that the individual coefficients associated with the IE solution are estimable in the sense that, for example, the age1 coefficient in the IE solution is an unbiased estimate of the age1 effect for the parameters that generated the outcome data. One nice feature of the *l'sv* procedure is that by testing one linear combination at a time, the researcher's attention is focused on what function is estimable.

---

[*] The other "meaningful" estimable functions represented by the rows are those for age 3, period 3, and cohort 5. These effects for these coefficients (as well as for the intercept) are estimable using any of the just identified constraints. For example, they are the same for the IE constraint as they are for the age1 = age2 constraint.

4.4 Some Examples of Estimable Functions Derived Using the *l'sv* Approach

4.4.1 Effect Coefficients

Some individual effect coefficients in the APC multiple classification model are estimable. Keeping in mind that *sv* differentiates the various solutions on the line of solutions (the best fitting solutions for both OLS and generalized linear models); we examine the individual null vector entries that correspond to each of the effect coefficients. If the null vector entry is zero, then for any of the constrained solutions, the parameter estimate corresponding to that null vector entry is invariant across all of the solutions including the solution that generated the outcome values. Let v_i represent the *i*th element of the null vector and b_i represent the *i*th element of the solution vector, then if $v_i = 0$, $b_i + sv_i = b_i$ no matter what the value of *s*. With effect coding, the intercept is always estimable and the middle parameters for age, period, and cohort are estimable if there is an odd number categories associated with the factor. These estimable functions were noted by Jagodzinski (1984) but derived differently.

For the sake of concreteness, Table 4.1 provides the null vectors for three situations: a 5×5 age–period matrix, a 4×4 age–period matrix, and a 4×5 age–period matrix. The null vector elements are in regular font and the "extended null vector" elements are italicized. The extended null vector elements represent the reference categories and are the implied extension given the other null vector elements. They are useful in extending the range of the estimable functions that are derived.[*] Examining the null vector elements for the 5×5 age–period case, the intercept, age 3, period 3, and cohort 5 coefficients are all estimable. These estimable functions are not very helpful. They are similar to the estimable coefficients when dummy variable coding is used; in that situation the reference categories are estimable, since they are coded in such a way as to generate a solution of zero across any constraint.

4.4.2 Second Differences

Second differences can be used to show the increase or decrease in the rate of change in age coefficients, period coefficients, and cohort coefficients. These second differences are estimable. Here I will not use the shortcut that if $l'v = 0$,

---

[*] These elements are the null vector elements of an *X*-matrix that contains columns for all of the independent variables—the *X*-matrix without having eliminated columns for the reference categories. If this matrix is labeled X^* and the extended null vector v^*, then $X^*v^* = 0$. This is why, as shown later, the extended null vector "works" for the coefficients associated with the reference categories.

TABLE 4.1

Null and Extended Null Vectors for Three Different Age–Period Tables

Effect Coefficients	5 × 5 Null Vector	4 × 4 Null Vector	4 × 5 Null Vector
		Dimensions of Age–Period Table	
Intercept	0	0	0
age 1	-2	-1.5	-1.5
age 2	-1	-0.5	-0.5
age 3	0	0.5	0.5
age 4	1	1.5	1.5
age 5	2		
period 1	2	1.5	2
period 2	1	0.5	1
period 3	0	-0.5	0
period 4	-1	-1.5	-1
period 5	-2		-2
cohort 1	-4	-3	-3.5
cohort 2	-3	-2	-2.5
cohort 3	-2	-1	-1.5
cohort 4	-1	0	-0.5
cohort 5	0	1	0.5
cohort 6	1	2	1.5
cohort 7	2	3	2.5
cohort 8	3		3.5
cohort 9	4		

Note: The extended null vector elements are in italics.

$l'sv = 0$ for all values of s, but instead will "deal with s explicitly." The reason for this is to provide an introduction to this method before encountering some derivations where this method is the easiest to use conceptually.

Let v_{ia} represent the elements of the extended null vector that correspond to the age effects: a_i ($i = 1$ to I). Note that the coding for the extended null vector for the age elements is linear and the intervals are equal (coded as an interval-level variable). Because of this the second differences for the age effects are invariant to the constraint used to solve the APC model. Consider the first three age effects; we can write the second difference for the age coefficients for the original solution as $(a_3 - a_2) - (a_2 - a_1) = a_1 - 2a_2 + a_3$. Next consider a different solution on the line of solutions with the scalar value s. The second difference for this new solution is $[(a_3 + sv_{3a}) - (a_2 + sv_{2a})] - [(a_2 + sv_{2a}) + (a_1 + sv_{1a})] = (a_1 + sv_{1a}) - 2(a_2 + sv_{2a}) + (a_3 + sv_{3a}) = a_1 - 2a_2 + a_3 + (sv_{1a} - 2sv_{2a} + sv_{3a})$, where v_{ia} is the ith age element of the null vector. Since v_{ia} is coded as a linear equal interval variable, $(sv_{1a} - 2sv_{2a} + sv_{3a}) = 0$, so that the second difference for any new solution is $(a_1 - 2a_2 + a_3)$, which is identical to the second difference for the original solution. Concretely, given the equal intervals between the elements of the null vector, the values for the first three age elements of sv_{ia} might be $sv_{1a} = 8$, $sv_{2a} = 6$, and $sv_{3a} = 4$, then the difference between the original and the new solution would be $+8 - (2 \times 6) + 4 = 0$.

To generalize this result, change the notation for a to a_i, a_{i+1}, and a_{i+2} and for v to v_{ia}, $v_{(i+1)a}$, and $v_{(i+2)a}$, and proceed with the aforementioned steps. One can only calculate $I - 2$ second differences for the age coefficients. Using the same procedure, the second differences for periods $(p_{j+2} - p_{j+1}) - (p_{j+1} - p_j)$ for $j = 1$ to $J - 2$ are estimable for $J - 2$ second differences, and the second differences for cohorts $(c_{k+2} - c_{k+1}) - (c_{k+1} - c_k)$ for $k = 1$ to $K - 2$ are estimable for $K - 2$ second differences.

4.4.3 Relationships between Slopes

Much can be learned about the relationships between the slopes of the age, period, and cohort coefficients based on different solutions by concentrating on sv.[*] Note that in Table 4.1 the v_{ia} *increase* linearly with equal intervals between the consecutive values of v_{ia}; the v_{jp} *decrease* linearly with equal intervals between the values of v_{jp}, and those intervals are the same in absolute value as those for v_{ia}; and the v_{kc} *increase* linearly with equal intervals between their values and the intervals are the same in absolute value as for v_{ia} and v_{jp}.[†] To compare the slopes of the age-coefficients, period-coefficients, and cohort-coefficients for the original solution to those for a new solution, I compare the slopes for the original solution vector with those of the original solution vector to which sv has been added.

The effect of adding sv_{ia} to each of the a_i coefficients is to change the slope of age by $s(v_{2a} - v_{1a})$. The result is the same for the effect of adding sv_{jp} to each of the p_j coefficients and sv_{kc} to each of the c_k coefficients. That is, it changes the period slope by $s(v_{2p} - v_{1p})$ and the cohort slope by $s(v_{2c} - v_{1c})$.[‡] For the coding in Table 4.1, for a positive value of s it would increase the slope by s for the age components, decrease it by s for period, and increase the cohort slope by s. This convenient result occurs because the distance between adjacent values of the age null vector elements is one, the period null vector elements is one, and the cohort null vector elements is one. But in terms of the relationship between the slopes, it will not matter if the distances between adjacent values of the null vector elements are all .4, 1, or 2, or some other number. The value of s will change to compensate for the multiplicative change in the

---

[*] These slopes are based on regressing the coefficients for age, for period, and for cohorts on time. For example, we would find the slope for age coefficients by regressing the a_i (age coefficients) on the integers 1, 2, ..., I.

[†] The null vector is unique up to multiplication by a scalar. If the scalar were negative, the direction of the slope would change. I will refer to the sign of increase or decrease being opposite for age and period, and period and cohort, and the same for age and cohort.

[‡] I write $s(v_{2a} - v_{1a})$ rather than $s(v_{(i+1)a} - v_{ia})$, since all of these intervals are equal and of the same sign; this could also be done for periods and cohorts. It seems simpler and understandable to use the notation $s(v_{2a} - v_{1a})$.

elements of the null vector. In any case, the slopes of age and period change by the same amount, but in opposite directions as do the slopes of period and cohort; while the slopes of age and cohort change by the same amount and in the same direction.

More formally, assume that the original solution has a trend of t_a for the age coefficients, t_p for the period coefficients, and t_c for the cohort coefficients. Since any new solution lies on the line of solutions, it differs from the original solution by sv. Specifically, the slopes for the new solution are $t_a + s(v_{2a} - v_{1a})$, $t_p + s(v_{2p} - v_{1p})$, and $t_c + s(v_{2c} - v_{1c})$. Although the null vector elements are only unique up to multiplication by a scalar, the distances between the age, period, and cohort null vector elements are all the same in absolute size: $|v_{2a} - v_{1a}| = |v_{2p} - v_{1p}| = |v_{2c} - v_{1c}|$. The sign of the differences for age and cohort are always the same, whereas the signs of the differences for age and period, and period and cohort are always opposite.

The estimable functions for the relationships among these slopes follow from these relationships. The sum of the age and period trends is estimable; this sum is the same no matter what the constraint. Note that $(v_{2a} - v_{1a})$ and $(v_{2p} - v_{1p})$ are of opposite sign, but of the same absolute value. Therefore, $t_a + t_p = (t_a + s(v_{2a} - v_{1a})) + (t_p + s(v_{2p} - v_{1p}))$, since $s(v_{2a} - v_{1a}) + s(v_{2p} - v_{1p}) = 0$. Using the same approach, we can show that $t_p + t_c$ is estimable: $t_p + t_c = (t_p + s(v_{2p} - v_{1p})) + t_c + s(v_{2c} - v_{1c}))$, since $s(v_{2p} - v_{1p}) + s(v_{2c} - v_{1c}) = 0$. For the two sets with null vector elements that are coded as trends in same directions (age and cohort), $t_a - t_c$ is an estimable function: $t_a - t_c = (t_a + s(v_{2a} - v_{1a})) - (t_c + s(v_{2c} - v_{1c}))$, since $s(v_{2a} - v_{1a}) - (v_{2c} - v_{1c}) = 0$. These relationships between the changes in slopes for age, period, and cohort are the same as those noted by Rodgers (1982), although derived in a different manner.

The results in this section allow us to derive the relationship between the slopes of age, period, and cohort. If we write the relationships for the sums of the trends equaling a constant across any of the constrained solutions as $t_a + t_p = k_1$, $t_p + t_c = k_2$, and that $t_a - t_c = k_3$, we see that $(t_a + t_p) - (t_a + t_c) = t_a - t_c = k_1 - k_2 = k_3$. Here a linear combination of estimable functions is used to derive an estimable function. These relationships between sums and differences of trends produce the same values no matter which just identifying constraint is used.

Holford (1985:834) shows "that the general form for the estimable relationships among the slopes (using my notation) is $d_1 t_a + d_2 t_p + (d_2 - d_1)t_c$. Using the *l'sv* method and the approach of this section, this relationship can be shown to hold for all of the constrained solutions. For the original solution we can write $d_1 t_a + d_2 t_p + (d_2 - d_1)t_c$, and for the new solution we can write $d_1(t_a + s(v_{2a} - v_{1a})) + d_2(t_p + s(v_{2p} - v_{1p})) + (d_2 - d_1)(t_c + s(v_{2c} - v_{1c}))$. Then, $d_1 t_a + d_2 t_p + (d_2 - d_1)t_c + [d_1 s(v_{2a} - v_{1a}) + d_2 s(v_{2p} - v_{1p}) + d_2 s(v_{2c} - v_{1c}) - d_1 s(v_{2c} - v_{1c})]$. Note that $s(v_{2a} - v_{1a})$ and $s(v_{2c} - v_{1c})$ are of the same sign and magnitude and $s(v_{2p} - v_{1p})$ is of opposite sign, but the same magnitude. The terms in square brackets sum to zero. This is the case for any choice of the values for d_1 and d_2. This function $d_1 t + d_2 t_p + (d_2 - d_1)t_c$ is estimable; it is the same for any of the just identified constrained solutions and for the parameters that generated the outcome values.

4.4.4 Change of Slope within Factors

Tarone and Chu (1996) demonstrated that the change in slopes within age groups, or within periods, or within cohorts is estimable. For example, if two sets of cohort coefficients are selected, the first from $k = 1$ to d and the second from $d + 1$ to K, we can calculate the linear trend for the first set (t_{c1}) and the linear trend for the second set (t_{c2}). For the original constrained solution the change in slopes is $t_{c2} - t_{c1}$. Changes in these trends from the first set of cohorts to the second set are the same for any of the constrained solutions. For a new solution, the trend for the first set of cohorts is $t_{c1} + s(v_{2c} - v_{1c})$ and for the second set of cohorts is $t_{c2} + s(v_{2c} - v_{1c})$. The change in slopes for this second solution is $t_{c2} - t_{c1} = (t_{c2} + s(v_{2c} - v_{1c})) - (t_{c1} + s(v_{2c} - v_{1c}))$, since $s(v_{2c} - v_{1c}) - s(v_{2c} - v_{1c}) = 0$. The change in trends is the same as for the original solution no matter what the value of s and, of course, for the generating parameters. The same approach can be used to show that the change in trends within periods and within age groups is the same for any of the constrained solutions. Using the $l's v$ approach, the estimability of changes in slopes can be shown to extend to more than two trends within cohorts or periods or age groups. We can also determine whether the trend in cohorts shifted more than the trend in periods.

4.4.5 Deviations from Linearity

In APC models it is the linear components that are not estimable and the nonlinear components of age, period, and cohort that are estimable (O'Brien 2011a), if we mean by this that the deviations of the age coefficients from the linear trend of the age coefficients, the deviations of the period coefficients from the linear trend of the period coefficients, and the deviations of the cohort coefficients from the linear trend of the cohort coefficients are invariant across the different solutions.[*] Again age coefficients for the original solution are represented as a_i and the elements from the extended null vector that corresponds to these elements as v_{ia}. The trend for the original solution is represented as t_a. With effect coding the values of the age coefficients (period coefficients and cohort coefficients) are centered on their mean effects. To find the predicted values of the age effect coefficients based on the trend, we can multiply the trend by the centered values (i_a), where before centering, i is a vector of integers $i = 1, 2, \ldots, I$. The predicted values of the age coefficients based on the linear effects of the original age coefficients are $t_a \cdot i_a$. The deviations of the age effects from linearity are $(a_i - t_a \cdot i_a)$.

---

[*] Holford (1983) proved that these deviations are estimable, but did so by recoding the variables for the X-matrix.

We can represent another solution for the age effects as $a_i + sv_{ia}$. The trend for the new age coefficients is $t_a + c(v_{2a} - v_{1a})$, and the predicted values for the new age coefficients based on the linear trend in the coefficients are $(t_a + s(v_{2a} - v_{1a})) \cdot i_a$. To show that the deviations of the age effects from the linear trend are estimable, note that the original deviations are $a_i - t_a \cdot i_a$ and the deviations for a different constrained solution are $[a_i + sv_{ia}] - [(t_a + s(v_{2a} - v_{1a})) \cdot i_a]$. The key to this proof is that $sv_{ia} = s(v_{2a} - v_{1a}) \cdot i_a$.[*] Therefore, $a_i - t_a \cdot i_a = [a_i + sv_{ia}] - [(t_a + s(v_{2a} - v_{1a})) \cdot i_a]$. The same method can be used to show that $p_j - t_p \cdot i_p$ and $c_k - t_c \cdot i_c$, the deviations of the period coefficients from the linear trend of the period coefficients and deviation of the cohort coefficients from the linear trend in the cohort coefficients are invariant across solutions. These deviations from the linear trends of age, period, and cohort are estimable.

4.4.6 Predicted Values of *y*

The predicted values of *y* are estimable; they are the same across all of the solutions and the same for the parameters that generated the outcome values. This is why the fit of APC models are the same for all of the constraints that just identify the rank deficient by one APC model. The prediction equation for the APC model tells us that the predicted values for each cell of the age–period table are the intercept plus the age effect for that cell plus the period effect for that cell plus the cohort effect for that cell.

No matter what the constraint, we will obtain the same solution for this predicted cell value because of an important relationship among the elements of *v*. We can write that relationship as $(v_0 + v_{ia} + v_{jp} + v_{kc} = 0)$, where v_0 represents the intercept, v_{ia} represents the *i*th age group, v_{jp} represents the *j*th period, and v_{kc} represents the *k*th cohort ($k = I - i + j$). For example, the oldest age group in the earliest period corresponds to the earliest cohort. Turning to Table 4.1 and the null vector for the 5×5 age–period matrix, we find that $v_0 = 0$; that for age 5, v_{ia} is 2; for period 1, v_{jp} is 2; and for cohort 1, v_{kc} is –4, and that $(v_0 + v_{ia} + v_{jp} + v_{kc}) = (0 + 2 + 2 - 4) = 0$. For any cell of the table, the null vector element corresponding to the intercept plus the null vector element corresponding to the age-effect plus the null vector element corresponding to period-effect plus the null vector element corresponding to the cohort effect is equal to zero. We write the original solution for the fitted value of the *ij*th cell of the age–period table as $\hat{y}_{ij} = int + a_i + p_j + c_k$. A different solution on the line of solutions can be written as $\hat{y}_{ij} = (int + sv_0) + (a_i + sv_{ia}) + p_j + sv_{jp}) + (c_k + sv_{kc})$. The new solution can be written as $\hat{y}_{ij} = int + a_i + p_j + c_k + s(v_0 + v_{ia} +$

---

[*] For example, in the 5 by 5 age-by-period case (Table 4.1) for the extended null vector: $v_{ia} = (-2, -1, 0, 1, 2)$ and $i_a = (-2, -1, 0, 1, 2)$ and $v_{2a} - v_{1a} = 1$; thus $sv_{ia} = s(v_{2a} - v_{1a}) \cdot i_2$; for periods the null vector elements are $v_{jp} = (2, 1, 0, -1, -2)$ while $i_p = (-2, -1, 0, 1, 2)$, but $v_{2p} - v_{1p} = -1$; thus, $sv_{jp} = s(v_{2p} - v_{1p}) \cdot i_p$. If we code the null vector as $-1/2$ times its coding in Table 4.1, it changes the elements of *v* to be one half as far apart and changes their signs, and *s* is adjusted to compensate for the change. This procedure above works with these changes.

$v_{jp} + v_{kc}$). The new solution equals the original solution: $\hat{y}_{ij} = int + a_i + p_j + c_k$, since $(v_0 + v_{ia} + v_{jp} + v_{kc}) = 0$. The estimated values of y_{ij} $(\hat{y}_{ij})$ are invariant and estimable.

4.5 Comments on the *l'sv* Approach

The derivations of important estimable functions in APC models are scattered throughout the literature and the methods used to establish these as estimable functions vary from simple algebra to a fairly elaborate recoding of the X-matrix to show that the function meets Searle's (1971) criterion. The approach outlined in this paper can be used to derive all of these estimable functions and others. It provides a necessary and sufficient condition for estimability.

For the estimable functions derived in this text, this criterion is straightforward for deriving *some* estimable functions, such as the one suggested by Jagodzinski (1984). In a 5×5 age–period table, if the age coefficient corresponding to a zero element in the null vector is the third age group element and the null vector elements are arranged as (intercept, age groups, periods, cohorts), then (0, 0, 0, 1, 0, ..., 0) is the appropriate linear combination(*l'*) and *l'sv* = 0 for any value of *s*. Another example is establishing that the second difference for age1, age2, and age3 is estimable (0, 1, –2, 1, 0, ..., 0). Several of the other estimable functions discussed in this chapter, however, even though based on the *l'sv* criterion, are difficult to place in a vector of numbers that can then be multiplied times *sv* to determine if the dot product is zero. We have shown how the *l'sv* criterion can be used in these more complex situations, such as the *l'sv* criterion of the effect coefficients for age groups, periods, and cohorts from the linear trends of the age coefficients, period coefficients, and cohort coefficients, or the difference of trends within age groups, periods, or cohorts.

Many important estimable functions have been presented, but we can derive other estimable functions. The sums of $a_i + p_j$ are invariant across solutions for $i = j$ when $I = J$. In any particular situation, such as our 5×5 age–period matrix, particular estimable functions may be found. For example, in the 5×5 situation the effect coefficient for cohort2 plus the effect coefficients for period1 plus period2 is invariant across solutions. This can be easily seen by examining the null vector for this 5×5 age–period matrix in Table 4.1. The *l'sv* approach is flexible for finding such "ad hoc" estimable functions when the dimensions of the age–period table differ, since the null vector is based on the dimensions of the age–period table. If one wants to know whether the change in trends within periods has been greater than the change in trends within cohorts, that function can be shown to be estimable using the approach outlined in this chapter.

The general method by which estimable functions are derived using the *l'sv* approach does not depend upon the way in which the independent variables are coded. For example, another common way to code the independent variables in the APC model is to use dummy variable coding. The solutions all lie on a line of solutions and when using *sv*, the null vector associated with the dummy variable coded X-matrix is used.[*]

4.6 Estimable Functions with Empirical Data

To illustrate the use of estimable functions, data from a recent study by Samuel Preston and Haidong Wang (2006) is used. The study focuses on changes in the gap between the life spans of men and women from 1948 to 2003. I will describe the study in greater detail in the next section when the focus is more directly substantive, but for now interest focuses on how the estimable functions derived earlier work with data. The data utilized come from Table 5 of Preston and Wang's paper (Table 4.2 in this chapter) and were not formally analyzed by them. The cells contain the differences in the lung cancer mortality rates for men and women per 100,000 (men's rates minus women's rates). In the analysis of this data these differences are logged. The oldest age group in the earliest period represents the earliest cohort and that

TABLE 4.2

Difference in Lung Cancer Death Rates for Men and Women per 100,000 Population

Age Group	Period											
	1948	1953	1958	1963	1968	1973	1978	1983	1988	1993	1998	2003
50–54	33.7	48.3	56.0	58.7	64.1	63.2	63.1	51.2	44.4	31.9	21.2	18.4
55–59	56.0	80.6	92.5	105.7	117.6	116.4	110.5	101.0	90.5	72.2	50.6	38.0
60–64	67.4	106.4	142.0	161.7	191.7	192.4	188.9	161.9	156.6	132.9	91.4	65.6
65–69	64.3	109.8	163.9	219.4	248.1	270.1	263.9	247.3	225.7	204.6	154.6	114.4
70–74	53.9	94.3	145.5	215.9	306.2	331.5	361.0	338.6	307.9	257.7	229.5	173.4
75–79	43.8	78.7	116.1	182.1	261.5	344.2	396.3	404.8	381.5	320.2	273.0	233.8
80–84	34.5	62.1	88.7	137.3	187.4	282.6	382.7	411.0	421.1	385.9	311.9	262.5

Source: Data from Preston, S.H., and H. Wang, 2006, Sex mortality differences in the United States: The role of cohort smoking patterns, *Demography* 43:631–46, Table 5.

Note: The table is rearranged with age groups in the rows and periods in the columns.

---

[*] We can always derive the null vector from the eigenvector for the zero eigenvalue of the X-matrix for the APC model, although formulas for finding the null vector for both effect-coded and dummy-coded data are presented in Chapter 2.

cohort is labeled 1863–1867 by Preston and Wang. For this age, period, and cohort combination the gap was 34.5 deaths per 100,000. Given the setup of the table the cohorts are on the main diagonals.

The problem for the analyst, of course, is that although age groups, periods, and cohorts may all be related to these rates independently, we cannot uniquely estimate the independent effects of each of the age groups, periods, and cohorts: the APC model is not identified. The theme of this chapter is that although this is the case, some linear combinations of the parameters that generated the outcome data can be estimated and these may well be of value to the analyst.

Table 4.3 presents the constrained solutions under four different constraints age1 = age2, coh1 = coh2, the intrinsic estimator, and the zero linear trend for periods constraint (ZLT-period). The intrinsic estimator (Yang et al. 2004, 2008) is constrained to be perpendicular to the null vector, and the ZLT-period constraint (O'Brien 2011c) constrains the period coefficients to have a zero linear trend. Table 4.3 also presents the extended null vector for these data, the results for the estimable deviations from linearity, and estimable second differences. Although it is not immediately apparent from Table 4.3, all of these solutions lie on the line of solutions. If we add 0.2489 times the corresponding null vector element to the coefficients for age1 = age2 constrained solution in Table 4.3, we obtain the constrained solution using the coh1 = coh2 constraint. That is, $b_{c1=c2} = b_{a1=a2} + sv$, where $s = 0.2489$. The same procedure works for moving from the age1 = age2 constrained solution to the intrinsic estimator solution using $s = 0.5323$ and from the age1 = age2 constrained solution to the constrained solution for the ZLT for periods constraint ($s = 0.5999$).

More apparent in Table 4.3 is that no matter what the solution, the intercept coefficients are the same (4.640) as are the coefficients for age 65–69 (0.205). In these cases the corresponding null vector element is zero, so these coefficients are the same across all of the constrained solutions. Note that otherwise the individual age, period, and cohort coefficients are different, sometimes quite different across the various constrained solutions.

In these models the trends for the age coefficients, the period coefficients, and the cohort coefficients are not identified (O'Brien 2011b), except in the narrow sense that they are identified given a particular constraint. If we could establish the trend of one of these sets of coefficients, we could identify the other effects in the model. That, however, is not possible without a constraint. But in the section on slopes, the $l'sv$ approach indicated that the sums and differences of specific trends are estimable in certain cases. That is, the sum of the age and period trends is estimable ($t_a + t_p$), the sum of the period and cohort trends is estimable ($t_p + t_c$), and the age trend minus the cohort trend is estimable ($t_a - t_c$). This is demonstrated in the bottom section of Table 4.3, where we see that no matter which constraint is used

TABLE 4.3

OLS Regression Results Using Logged Differences between Men and Women in the Rates of Lung Cancer Mortality

	age1 = age2	coh1 = coh2	Intrinsic Estimator	ZLT– Period	Extended Null Vector	Deviations from Linearity	Second Differences
intercept	4.640	4.640	4.640	4.640	0.000		
50–54	0.603	–0.143	–0.993	–1.196	–3.000	–0.276	
55–59	0.603	0.106	–0.461	–0.596	–2.000	0.017	
60–64	0.463	0.214	–0.069	–0.137	–1.000	0.170	–0.140
65–69	0.205	0.205	0.205	0.205	0.000	0.205	–0.117
70–74	–0.149	0.099	0.383	0.450	1.000	0.144	–0.097
75–79	–0.602	–0.104	0.463	0.598	2.000	–0.016	–0.097
80–84	–1.124	-0.378	0.473	0.675	3.000	–0.245	–0.070
1948	–3.575	–2.206	–0.647	–0.275	5.500	–6.874	
1953	–2.773	–1.653	–0.378	–0.074	4.500	–5.473	
1958	–2.116	–1.245	–0.253	–0.017	3.500	–4.216	–0.145
1963	–1.448	–0.826	–0.117	0.052	2.500	–2.948	0.011
1968	–0.775	–0.402	0.024	0.125	1.500	–1.675	0.005
1973	–0.140	–0.015	0.126	0.160	0.500	–0.440	–0.038
1978	0.487	0.363	0.221	0.187	–0.500	0.787	–0.008
1983	1.031	0.657	0.232	0.131	–1.500	1.931	–0.084
1988	1.607	0.985	0.276	0.107	–2.500	3.107	0.033
1993	2.115	1.244	0.252	0.015	–3.500	4.215	–0.069
1998	2.554	1.435	0.159	–0.145	–4.500	5.254	–0.068
2003	3.032	1.664	0.105	–0.267	–5.500	6.332	0.038
1863–67	3.600	1.485	–0.925	–1.499	–8.500	–0.983	
1868–72	3.351	1.485	–0.641	–1.148	–7.500	–0.693	
1873–77	3.086	1.468	–0.374	–0.813	–6.500	–0.419	–0.016
1878–82	2.852	1.483	–0.076	–0.447	–5.500	–0.113	0.032
1883–87	2.604	1.484	0.209	–0.095	–4.500	0.178	–0.014
1888–92	2.328	1.457	0.465	0.228	–3.500	0.441	–0.028
1893–97	1.946	1.324	0.616	0.447	–2.500	0.599	–0.105
1898–02	1.437	1.064	0.639	0.538	–1.500	0.629	–0.128
1903–07	0.907	0.783	0.641	0.607	–0.500	0.637	–0.021
1908–12	0.292	0.416	0.558	0.592	0.500	0.561	–0.085
1913–17	–0.350	0.023	0.448	0.550	1.500	0.459	–0.026
1918–22	–1.011	–0.389	0.320	0.488	2.500	0.337	–0.020
1923–27	–1.628	–0.757	0.235	0.472	3.500	0.259	0.045
1928–32	–2.348	–1.228	0.048	0.352	4.500	0.078	–0.103
1933–37	–3.104	–1.736	–0.177	0.195	5.500	–0.139	–0.036
1938–42	–3.907	–2.290	–0.447	–0.008	6.500	–0.403	–0.047
1943–47	–4.691	–2.825	–0.699	–0.192	7.500	–0.647	0.019
1948–52	–5.364	–3.248	–0.839	–0.265	8.500	–0.780	0.111

TABLE 4.3 (continued)

OLS Regression Results Using Logged Differences between Men and Women
in the Rates of Lung Cancer Mortality

	age1 = age2	coh1 = coh2	Intrinsic Estimator	ZLT– Period
	Trends			
Age	−0.293	−0.044	0.239	0.307
Period	0.600	0.351	0.068	0.000
Cohort	−0.539	−0.290	−0.007	0.061
Age + Period	0.307	0.307	0.307	0.307
Period + Cohort	0.061	0.061	0.061	0.061
Age − Cohort	0.246	0.246	0.246	0.246

Note: The data are from Table 4.2.

$(t_a + t_p) = 0.307$, $(t_p + t_c) = 0.061$, and $(t_a - t_c) = 0.246$. Although the trends are different depending upon the constraint used, these sums and differences are the same.

The deviations of the age coefficients from their linear trend are presented in Table 4.3 and are the same no matter which constraint is used to solve the APC model. For example, these deviations from linearity (−0.276, 0.017, 0.170, 0.205, 0.144, −0.016, −0.245) for age 50–54 to age 80–84 are the same no matter what constraint is used to obtain the solution. The second differences (differences of differences) are equal for each of the constraints. For the second difference for (age3 − 2 × age2 + age1) using the age1 = age2 constraint is −0.140 = [+(0.463) − 2 × (0.603) + (0.603)] and for the IE constraint for the same linear combination it is −0.140 [= (−0.069 − 2 × (−0.461) + (−0.993)]. These second differences are equal, as they must be for estimable functions. Table 4.3 contains the second differences for the age, period, and cohort coefficients in the final column.

A researcher probably would not want to test the change in the trend within ages, since there are so few age coefficients. For substantive reasons (described in the next section), we focus on changes in trends within cohorts. We split the cohort coefficients into two groups 1863–1867 through 1898–1902 and 1903–1907 through 1948–1952. The change in slope (most recent cohort trend minus the earlier cohort trend), which is an estimable function and the same no matter what constrained solution we use, is −.410 (this is in terms of the trends in the logged difference in rates). The data show a strong difference in the trends of the cohort effects for the earlier and more recent cohorts: the more recent set of cohorts has a trend that is less positive than the earlier set of cohorts.

The predicted values of y (predicted logged cell rates for the age-period table) are the same no matter what the constraint used to obtain the solution. As an example, the cell that corresponds to those 50–54 years old in 1948 (who therefore are part of the 1893–1897 cohort) is used. The predicted value for this cell is the intercept + age50–54 + period1948 + cohort1893–1897. For the age1 = age2 constraint, this is 4.640 + 0.630 – 3.575 + 1.946 = 3.614 and for the cohort1 = cohort2 constraint, the linear combination is 4.640 – 0.143 – 2.206 + 1.324 = 3.615. The value is the same (within rounding error) no matter which of the constrained results are used. Since the dependent variable in our analysis is logged, we can exponentiate this value to obtain the estimated gap between men and women in the number of deaths per 100,000 in this cell, which is 37.11. In Table 4.2 we see that the observed value is 33.7 per 100,000.

4.7 More Substantive Examination of Differences of Male and Female Lung Cancer Mortality Rates

As noted in the previous section, the data in Table 4.2 come from a study by Preston and Wang (2006). That data focus on differences in mortality rates between men and women. In the main part of their study, Preston and Wang examine differences in the rates of mortality in the United States between men and women, and how they have changed over time for different age groups. The data show that the gap between the life spans of men and women has decreased in recent periods, and Preston and Wang argue convincingly that this has occurred, in large part, because the gap in smoking between men and women in various cohorts has been decreasing. They report evidence showing that there was a 10.7 year difference in the estimated number of years spent as a smoker before the age of 40 for cohort members born between 1885 and 1889. This increased to 13.5 years for those born between 1895 and 1899. There has been a monotonic decrease in this gap from that cohort through the cohort born between 1950 and 1954.

Like tuberculosis, which was discussed in conjunction with Frost's (1939) study, the effects of smoking on lung cancer rates may appear long after exposure to the disease-causing "substance." As noted in the previous section, the data in Table 4.2 is a portion of their data. It is a portion that they did not analyze in a formal manner, but it is used now to demonstrate the usefulness of estimable functions in a specific substantive context.[*]

Given their discussion of the literature, which emphasizes a decreasing gap between the smoking behavior of men and women for the cohorts born

_____

[*] The data appear in Table 5 of their paper; they obtained them from the National Center for Health Statistics.

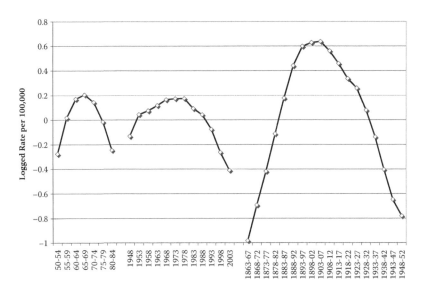

FIGURE 4.1
Deviations from linearity for the logged differences between male and female mortality rates due to lung cancer.

after 1900, we would expect, at a minimum, that the rate of increase in the gap between men and women in terms of lung cancer mortality would decrease for those born after 1900. If smoking were the predominant factor creating the gap, we would expect the gap in lung cancer mortality to decrease after 1900. This leads us to expect that deviations of the cohort effect from linearity will follow an inverted U-shaped pattern and that the change in the slope of the cohort effects will be negative (at least for the trends before and after 1900). These patterns would be consistent with Preston and Wang's theory.

The calculated cohort effect deviations from linearity are reported in Table 4.3 and graphed in Figure 4.1. These cohort deviations have the inverted U-shape that we would expect, if the "rate of increase" in the gap between the lung cancer mortality rates for men and women generally decreased across cohorts.

The reason for this cautious language about the "rate of increase" is that even with this inverted U-shaped curve for the deviations from linearity, one can find a constrained solution in which the gap increases across cohorts, but that increase is at a decreasing rate. We also expect the slope to be less positive for the more recent cohorts than for the earlier cohorts. The change of slope for cohorts is an estimable function. With the substantive theory from Preston and Wang's (2006) article and their data on years of smoking before the age of 40, one would expect the trend in the cohort effects on the gap between the lung cancer mortality rates for men and women to be more positive (less negative) for the cohorts born from 1863–1867 through

1898–1902 and less positive (more negative) for those cohort born from 1903–1907 through 1948–1952. The change in slope for these two sets of cohort is −.410. The data show a strong difference in the trends of the cohort effects for the earlier and more recent cohorts with the earlier cohorts being more positive (less negative) than the more recent cohorts. The slope for the earlier cohorts is statistically significantly different from the slope for the more recent cohorts ($p < .001$).

Examining Figure 4.1 further, there appears to be a fairly smooth curvilinear relationship between period deviations from their linear trend and between age deviations from their linear trend and the gap between lung cancer mortality for men and women. But just as for cohorts, we cannot say that this relationship is an inverted U-shape for the age and period effects themselves, since their linear trend components have been removed.

4.8 Conclusions

In its classical form, the unconstrained APC model is unidentified, since the design matrix (X) is rank deficient by one. There are an infinite number of solutions for the effect coefficients that fit the outcome data equally well. We can, however, find *a* solution to the APC model by placing a single constraint on the coefficients. This solution provides the best estimates of the cell values for the APC model as does any other constrained solution.

Although such a constraint results in the best fitting solutions for the predicted values of the dependent variable, the solutions for the effect coefficients vary with the constraint. Despite this we can find unique estimates of some linear combinations of these effect coefficients. These "estimable functions" are the same no matter which of the just identified linear constraints are used to find a solution. They are invariant across the solutions. Crucial for those researchers interested in substantive issues, these estimable functions are unbiased estimates of these linear combinations for the parameters that generated the outcome variables. Like all of the other best fitting solutions, the solution for the parameters that generated the outcome data must lie on the line of solutions.

The approach presented in this chapter for establishing the linear combinations that are estimable functions is based on the fact that all of the constrained solutions lie on the line of solutions: $b_c^0 = b_{c1}^0 + sv$. This method unifies the derivation of estimable functions and can be used with ordinary least squares and generalized linear models.

As an example of the utility of estimable functions, this chapter used data from Preston and Wang (2006) to show how the implications of their theory, which attributes part of the gap between the lung cancer mortality rates of men and women to cohort effects, can be tested with estimable functions. We can test such implications, even though we cannot estimate uniquely the age, period, and cohort effect coefficients, because we can estimate uniquely whether there is a change in the slope for cohorts between different sets of cohorts or whether the rate of change in cohort effects is increasing or decreasing.

The approach described in this chapter is not limited to APC models. For any rank deficient by one X-matrix the least squares and the generalized linear model solutions lie on a line of solutions, and the null vector supplies the direction of that line. For any rank deficient by two X-matrices the solutions lie on a plane of solutions and the direction of that plane is supplied by the space associated with the null space, which in this case will be of two dimensions. This approach can be extended to any number of null space dimensions.* The next chapter presents APC methods that are based on variance decomposition. For one of these approaches, the APC ANOVA approach, the decomposition is based on estimable functions.

Appendix 4.1

(See Table A4.1.1.)

---

* For a rank deficient by two matrix the solutions lie on a plane that is parallel to the null space. The plane of solutions is $b_c^0 = b_{c1}^0 + s_1 v_1 + s_2 v_2$ (O'Brien 2012), where v_1 and v_2 are linearly independent null vectors.

TABLE A4.1.1

Generalized Inverse for Solving the IE When the Age–Period Table Is 5×5

$I - \beta_0\beta_0'$

	Intercept	a1ie	a2ie	a3ie	a4ie	p1ie	p2ie	p3ie	p4ie	c1ie	c2ie	c3ie	c4ie	c5ie	c6ie	c7ie	c8ie	v
Intercept	1.0000	0.0000	0.0000	0.0000	0.0000	0.0000	0.0000	0.0000	0.0000	0.0000	0.0000	0.0000	0.0000	0.0000	0.0000	0.0000	0.0000	0.0000
a1ie	0.0000	0.9286	-0.0357	0.0000	0.0357	0.0714	0.0357	0.0000	-0.0357	-0.1429	-0.1071	-0.0714	-0.0357	0.0000	0.0357	0.0714	0.1071	-0.2673
a2ie	0.0000	-0.0357	0.9821	0.0000	0.0179	0.0357	0.0179	0.0000	-0.0179	-0.0714	-0.0536	-0.0357	-0.0179	0.0000	0.0179	0.0357	0.0536	-0.336
a3ie	0.0000	0.0000	0.0000	1.0000	0.0000	0.0000	0.0000	0.0000	0.0000	0.0000	0.0000	0.0000	0.0000	0.0000	0.0000	0.0000	0.0000	0.0000
a4ie	0.0000	0.0357	0.0179	0.0000	0.9821	-0.0357	-0.0179	0.0000	0.0179	0.0714	0.0536	0.0357	0.0179	0.0000	-0.0179	-0.0357	-0.0536	0.336
p1ie	0.0000	0.0714	0.0357	0.0000	-0.0357	0.9286	-0.0357	0.0000	0.0357	0.1429	0.1071	0.0714	0.0357	0.0000	-0.0357	-0.0714	-0.1071	0.673
p2ie	0.0000	0.0357	0.0179	0.0000	-0.0179	-0.0357	0.9821	0.0000	0.0179	0.0714	0.0536	0.0357	0.0179	0.0000	-0.0179	-0.0357	-0.0536	0.336
p3ie	0.0000	0.0000	0.0000	0.0000	0.0000	0.0000	0.0000	1.0000	0.0000	0.0000	0.0000	0.0000	0.0000	0.0000	0.0000	0.0000	0.0000	0.000
p4ie	0.0000	-0.0357	-0.0179	0.0000	0.0179	0.0357	0.0179	0.0000	0.9821	-0.0714	-0.0536	-0.0357	-0.0179	0.0000	0.0179	0.0357	0.0536	-0.336
c1ie	0.0000	-0.1429	-0.0714	0.0000	0.0714	0.1429	0.0714	0.0000	-0.0714	0.7143	-0.2143	-0.1429	-0.0714	0.0000	0.0714	0.1429	0.2143	-0.545
c2ie	0.0000	-0.1071	-0.0536	0.0000	0.0536	0.1071	0.0536	0.0000	-0.0536	-0.2143	0.8393	-0.1071	-0.0536	0.0000	0.0536	0.1071	0.1607	-0.409
c3ie	0.0000	-0.0714	-0.0357	0.0000	0.0357	0.0714	0.0357	0.0000	-0.0357	-0.1429	-0.1071	0.9286	-0.0357	0.0000	0.0357	0.0714	0.1071	-0.273
c4ie	0.0000	-0.0357	-0.0179	0.0000	0.0179	0.0357	0.0179	0.0000	-0.0179	-0.0714	-0.0536	-0.0357	0.9821	0.0000	0.0179	0.0357	0.0536	-0.136
c5ie	0.0000	0.0000	0.0000	0.0000	0.0000	0.0000	0.0000	0.0000	0.0000	0.0000	0.0000	0.0000	0.0000	1.0000	0.0000	0.0000	0.0000	0.000
c6ie	0.0000	0.0357	0.0179	0.0000	-0.0179	-0.0357	-0.0179	0.0000	0.0179	0.0714	0.0536	0.0357	0.0179	0.0000	0.9821	-0.0357	-0.0536	0.136
c7ie	0.0000	0.0714	0.0357	0.0000	-0.0357	-0.0714	-0.0357	0.0000	0.0357	0.1429	0.1071	0.0714	0.0357	0.0000	-0.0357	0.9286	-0.1071	0.2673
c8ie	0.0000	0.1071	0.0536	0.0000	-0.0536	-0.1071	-0.0536	0.0000	0.0536	0.2143	0.1607	0.1071	0.0536	0.0000	-0.0536	-0.1071	0.8393	0.409

References

Clayton, D., and E. Schifflers. 1987. Models for temporal variation in cancer rates II: Age-period-cohort models. *Statistics in Medicine* 6:468–81.

Frost, W.H. 1939. The age selection of mortality from tuberculosis in successive decades. *American Journal of Hygiene* 30:91–96.

Holford, T.R. 1983. The estimation of age, period, and cohort effects for vital rates. *Biometrics* 39:311–24.

Holford, T.R. 1985. An alternative approach to statistical age-period-cohort analysis. *Journal of Chronic Disease* 38:831–6.

Holford, T.R. 1991. Understanding the effects of age, period, and cohort on incidence and mortality rates. *Annual Review of Public Health* 12:425–57.

Holford, T.R. 2005. Age-period-cohort analysis. In *Encyclopedia of Biostatistics* (2nd edition), eds. P. Armitage and T. Colton, 105–23. Chichester, West Sussex, UK: John Wiley & Sons.

Jagodzinski, W. 1984. Identification of parameters in cohort models. *Sociological Methods & Research* 12:375–98.

Kupper, L.L., J.M. Janis, A. Karmous, and B.G. Greenberg. 1985. Statistical age-period-cohort analysis: A review and critique. *Journal of Chronic Disease* 38:811–30.

Mason, K.O., W.M. Mason, H.H. Winsborough, and K.W. Poole. 1973. Some methodological issues in cohort analysis of archival data. *American Sociological Review* 38:242–58.

O'Brien, R.M. 2011a. The age-period-cohort conundrum as two fundamental problems. *Quality & Quantity* 45:1429–44.

O'Brien, R.M. 2011b. Constrained estimators and age-period-cohort models. *Sociological Methods & Research* 40:419–52.

O'Brien, R.M. 2011c. Intrinsic estimators as constrained estimators in age-period-cohort accounting models. *Sociological Methods & Research* 40:467–70.

O'Brien, R.M. 2014. Estimable functions of age-period-cohort models: A unified approach. *Quality and Quantity* 48:457–474.

O'Brien R.M. 2012. Visualizing rank deficient models: A row equation geometry of rank deficient matrices and constrained-regression. *PLoS ONE* 7(6): e38923 doi:10.1371/journal.pone.0038923.

O'Brien, R.M., and J. Stockard 2009. Can cohort replacement explain changes in the relationship between age and homicide offending? *Journal of Quantitative Criminology* 25:79–101.

Preston, S.H., and H. Wang. 2006. Sex mortality differences in the United States: The role of cohort smoking patterns. *Demography* 43:631–46.

Robertson, C., S. Gandini, and P. Boyle. 1999. Age-period-cohort models: A comparative study of available methodologies. *Journal of Clinical Epidemiology* 52:569–83.

Rodgers, W.L. 1982. Estimable functions of age, period, and cohort effects. *American Sociological Review* 47:774–87.

Searle, S.R. 1971. *Linear Models.* New York: John Wiley & Sons.

Tarone, R.E., and K.C. Chu. 1996. Evaluation of birth cohort patterns in population disease rates. *American Journal of Epidemiology,* 143:85–91.

Yang, Y., W.J. Fu, and K.C. Land 2004. A methodological comparison of age-period-cohort models: Intrinsic estimator and conventional generalized linear models. In *Sociological Methodology*, ed. R.M. Stolzenberg, 75–110. Oxford: Basil Blackwell.

Yang, Y., and K.C. Land. 2013. *Age-Period-Cohort Analysis: New Models, Methods, and Empirical Applications*. Boca Raton, FL: Chapman & Hall.

Yang, Y., S. Schulhofer-Wohl, W.J. Fu, and K.C. Land. 2008. The intrinsic estimator for age-period-cohort analysis: What it is and how to use it. *American Journal of Sociology* 113:1697–736.

5

Partitioning the Variance in Age–Period–Cohort (APC) Models

Thus, I simply note that when one changes a model via random effects ... without strong prior information, one is still changing the model by fiat.

S.E. Fienberg (2013:1983)

5.1 Introduction

Variance decomposition using the analysis of variance is an estimable function and could have been placed in the previous chapter that focuses on estimable functions. It appears here, however, because it is closely related to the age–period–cohort mixed model (APCMM) method of determining the variance associated with random factors that is not an estimable function. Both the analysis of variance approach and the APCMM approach are excellent ways to wrest information about the unique effects of ages, periods, and cohorts from APC data. The APCMM is also related to the hierarchical age–period–cohort (HAPC) model of Yang and Land (2006). I will mention several of these relationships in this chapter that should help readers gauge some of the advantages and limits of these approaches.

Because of the linear dependency between the three factors—ages, periods, and cohorts—if only two of the factors are entered into a model, they will take credit for any linear trends in the third factor. If the two factors are age and period, for example, what remains for the cohort factor to explain are the deviations of the cohort coefficients from linearity. In Chapter 4 these deviations from linearity were shown to be estimable. The variance partitioning approach used in the first section of this chapter assesses the variance of these deviations. Using cohorts as an example, if the deviations of the cohort effects from linearity are statistically significant, then cohorts are uniquely associated with some of the variance in the outcome variable after controlling for age and period effects. Since these deviations from linearity are estimable, they are true for all constrained models and for the parameters that generated the outcome values.

Using this variance decomposition technique, however, the researcher cannot assess the amount of variance in the outcome variable that is due to the linear trend component for the factor that is entered into the model last. Additionally, since the two factors that are introduced first "absorb" any linear effects of the third factor, estimates of their parameters are not unbiased estimates of the effects of the corresponding data-generating parameters. This is a recurring problem: the trends of the age, period, and cohort effects cannot be identified without some outside information, and if we use outside information, the estimates are no better than that information. These methods, however, can be used to assess the nonlinear effects of these three factors and, for that purpose, can be used with confidence.

In the next two sections of this chapter two ways in which this variance partitioning can be accomplished are presented: the APC analysis of variance (ANOVA) approach (O'Brien and Stockard 2009) and the APCMM approach (O'Brien, Hudson, and Stockard 2008). Then an approach using data at both the individual level and aggregate level in the same model is described: the HAPC approach of Yang and Land (2006). This approach is somewhat outside of the scope of this book, which focuses on aggregate (macrodata) approaches, but it is closely related to the two other aggregate-level approaches described in this chapter. Examining the APC ANOVA and APCMM approaches will shed light on why the HAPC approach works in terms of being identified. The APC ANOVA and APCMM approaches to variance decomposition produce a "sufficient condition" for determining whether the age effects, period effects, and cohort effects contribute (statistically significantly) to the fit of the model.

5.2 Age–Period–Cohort Analysis of Variance (APC ANOVA) Approach to Attributing Variance

The ANOVA approach is most simply described in the case of an APC model that uses ordinary least squares (OLS), since that is the context in which ANOVA is typically presented. Chapters 2 and 4 show that if single constraints are placed on the APC coefficients the various constrained solutions will produce identical predicted values for the dependent variable. These are the predicted values that minimize the sum of the squared deviations of the observed y values from their predicted values. The R^2-value for the full APC model is $R^2_{y_{apc}}$. Here, $R^2_{y_{apc}}$ is the multiple correlation coefficient squared for the APC model with a single constraint. R^2_{ap} is the R^2-value for the model that contains the age and period categorical variables. The R^2-values indicate the proportion of the total variance in the outcome variable that is associated with each of these models.

The model that contains the categorically coded variables for age and period effects, accounts for the linear effects of cohorts as well as the linear and nonlinear effects of age and period. This occurs because the linear trends in age, period, and cohort are linearly dependent. The proportion of the variance in the outcome variable uniquely attributable to cohorts is $R^2_{diff} = R^2_{apc} - R^2_{ap}$. In the context of APC models with the linear dependency between the three factors, this unique proportion of the variance associated with cohorts captures the nonlinear effects of cohorts. A similar process can be used to calculate the unique period effects and age effects.

This formulation extends to generalized linear models, albeit in a modified form, in terms of the comparative fit of different models. Comparative fit for the different models is based on the likelihood ratio chi-square statistic. This statistic can be written as $-2 \times$ (Log-likelihood function for the reduced model $-$ Log-likelihood function for the fuller model). For example, to assess whether the full model (with one constraint) that includes the intercept and the age, period, and cohort factor fits the data significantly better than a model that contains only the intercept, we calculate the difference between the log-likelihoods, that for the model containing only the intercept minus that for the model containing the intercept and the three factors (with a single constraint), and multiply this difference by -2. The result is an approximate chi-square value with degrees of freedom equal to the difference in number of independent variables in the fuller model minus the number of independent variables in the reduced model. Note the similarity to the R^2 measure that is based on the variance accounted for by a model that contains only the intercept versus a model that contains the intercept, and the age, period, and cohort factors (with a single constraint). Similarly, we can compare the fit of the model that contains the intercept and all three factors (with a single constraint) to that of the model that contains the intercept and only two of the factors by considering the three-factor model as the full model and the two-factor model as the reduced model and computing the likelihood ratio chi-square.[*] This is analogous to the difference in R^2 test for the OLS model. Information criteria such as the Bayesian information criterion (BIC) and the Akaike information criterion (AIC) can also be used to compare the fit of models. These take into consideration the number of cases and/or the number of parameter estimates in the models, analogous to the corrected value of R^2.

To demonstrate the ANOVA approach, we turn to the data on breast cancer (Clayton and Schifflers 1987:Table 1) used in Chapter 2 (Table 2.3). Analyses are performed using both OLS regression on the logged rates of breast cancer per 100,000 women and Poisson regression on the age–period-specific counts

---

[*] It is referred to as the likelihood ratio chi-square because its formula can be written as

$$-2ln\left[\frac{\text{likelihood of the reduced model}}{\text{likelihood of the full model}}\right].$$

of breast cancer using as an exposure rate the number of women in each of the age–period-specific categories (see Clayton and Schifflers 1987, for more details about the data). The following procedure is used to determine if the unique effects of the nonlinear components of age are statistically significant using OLS regression. Run a regression analysis that includes all three factors (age, period, and cohort) with one of the nonreference categories for age omitted (in addition to omitting reference categories for age, period, and cohort). Excluding one extra age group category makes the model just identified and results in one of the infinite number of least squares solutions. It produces the least squares estimates of the predicted values of the dependent variable and thus the appropriate R^2 for the proportion of variance accounted for by age, period, and cohort. Run a model with only the period and cohort factors; that model accounts for the variance associated with these two factors and the variance associated with any linear trend associated with age. The difference in R^2 between the full model and the cohort–period model provides the proportion of the variance in the outcome variable uniquely associated with age groups.[*] This unique variance is that associated with the detrended age effects. One can follow the analogous procedures to determine the variances uniquely associated with period effects and cohort effects.

The same procedure is used with Poisson regression for testing the significance of the nonlinear components of age except that the test procedure uses the likelihood ratio chi-square test of the significance. Run a full model that eliminates one extra age effect (in addition to the reference categories) and a reduced model that eliminates the age factor entirely. This assures that the more restricted model that omits all of the ages is nested within the model that contains all but one age group (in addition to the age group used for a reference category). Then compare the full model with the reduced model using the likelihood ratio chi-square test. These comparisons can also be made using information criteria (BIC or AIC). To test the unique contribution to the fit of the model for periods and for cohorts one can use analogous procedures.

The results of these analyses appear in Table 5.1. Using OLS to analyze the logged age–period-specific rates of breast cancer, the results indicate that age, period, and cohort each account for a significant amount of unique variance in the logged breast cancer rates. After controlling for age and period, cohorts are associated with a unique percentage (.42%) of variance in breast cancer rates. After controlling for cohort and age effects, periods are associated with a unique percentage (0.12%) of the variance in breast cancer rates. After controlling for cohort and period effects, age groups are associated with a unique percentage (15.95%) of the variance in the breast cancer rates. Note this very strong unique relationship for ages. Even discounting any possible linear effects of age groups, they account for almost 16% of the

---

[*] I used Stata's "test" command to calculate the *F*-test of omitting all of the age variables from the equation for the full model (StataCorp 2013).

TABLE 5.1

Tests for the Unique Effects of Cohorts, Age, and Period after Controlling for the Other Two Factors

	OLS Regression of Logged Rates			
	Degrees of Freedom	P <	F	$R^2_{increment}$
Cohorts	F(13, 27)	0.0001	13.66	.0042
Periods	F(3,27)	0.0001	15.86	.0012
Ages	F(9,27)	0.0001	750.49	.1595

	Poisson Regression of Counts		
	Degrees of Freedom	P <	Chi-Square
Cohorts	Chi(13)	0.0001	186.8
Periods	Chi(3)	0.0001	55.53
Ages	Chi(9)	0.0001	3598.29

variance in the logged breast cancer rates. Each of these unique effects of cohorts, period, and ages is statistically significant at the .0001 level.

For Poisson regression the interpretation is not in terms of variance, instead it is in terms of the fit of the model as measured by the likelihood functions for the different models. In each case, the fit is significantly better (p < .0001) using the unique contributions of age, period, and cohort effects (in addition to that accounted for by the other two factors). Though not reported, BIC and the AIC each indicate that the model that includes ages, periods, and cohorts fits the data better than the models that leave out one of these factors. These information criteria take into account the sample size and the number of independent variables in the model. Note again that these results are based on estimable functions. They are the same for each of the constrained estimators that just identify the model, and they are the same for the generating parameters even though we do not know these parameters.* For the generating parameters there is a unique effect of cohorts, periods, and age groups in terms of variance accounted for in the OLS analysis and in terms of model fit in the Poisson analysis.

I want to emphasize the importance of this test strategy. It is a test that is sufficient for showing that a factor is statistically significantly related to age–period-specific rates in an APC model. So in this case, the significance tests indicate that the effects of age, the effects of period, and the effects of cohort are uniquely related to the outcome variable. These tests, however, are not a necessary condition for the factor to be related to the outcome variable. They test only the deviations from the linear trend of the factor and whether these deviations are related to the outcome variable. If they are not significantly related to the outcome variable, the factor's linear trend plus these deviations

---

* We note again that this assumes that the full APC model is the correct specification.

might well be significantly related to the outcome variable, but that trend is not estimable.

This model can be extended in additional ways. O'Brien and Stockard (2009) demonstrate that interactions can be added to the full model. For example, with the breast cancer data and with age1 omitted for identification, age2*per1 and age2*per4 interaction terms can be added to the model.[*] This is possible because these two interactions do not reintroduce the linear dependency between age, period, and cohort. In this case these two interactions are each statistically significant. Here, these interactions were chosen for a not totally justifiable reason (they fit large residuals), but in the empirical example at the end of this chapter interactions are selected for more substantive reasons. In that empirical example, I will also show how to use cohort characteristics in this context to determine how much of the variance due to cohorts can be accounted for by these particular cohort characteristics.

5.3 APC Mixed Model

In mixed models some of the variables are treated as fixed and others as random. The mixed model when ages and periods are treated as fixed effects and cohorts as random effects can be written as

$$y_{ijk} = \mu + \alpha_i + \pi_j + u_k + \epsilon_{ijk}. \tag{5.1}$$

In the age–period table, y_{ijk} is the dependent variable value for the ith age group and jth period with the corresponding kth cohort; μ is the intercept, α_i is the fixed effect for the ith age group, π_j is the fixed effect for the jth period, u_k represents the random effect for the kth cohort, and ϵ_{ijk} represents the random residual effect. For the fixed effects (ages and periods) one category serves as a reference category for each factor.

By modeling the cohorts as random effects, the APCMM provides estimates of the variation between cohorts while controlling for the effects of the age and period categories. No additional constraints need to be made for the model to be identified; those constraints are implicit in the model itself. For example, the random effects of cohort not only sum to zero, but that they have no linear trend across cohorts. I demonstrate this later, but first we note one extension to the APCMM that will be used later:

$$y_{ijk} = \mu + \alpha_i + \pi_j + b_k CohortCharacteristic + u_k + \epsilon_{ijk}. \tag{5.2}$$

---

[*] We obtain the same estimates for the two interactions using other constraints such as omitting cohort 1, even though, the coefficients for the age, period, and cohort effects differ because different constraints change the linear trends associated with age, period, and cohort coefficients.

That is, we can add one or more characteristics of cohorts to Equation (5.1). I introduce factor characteristics in Chapter 6; for now just consider them as measures associated with cohorts that may help account for differences between cohorts (for example, the average number of years spent smoking before the age of 35 for members of a cohort or the average number of years that cohort members spent in single-parent families when they were 0 to 12 years old). Adding one or more cohort characteristics to an age–period model will, in general, not result in a linear dependency. Note that in Equation (5.2) the random effects for cohorts can be included along with the cohort character-istic. This allows us to examine how these random effects are affected by adding cohort characteristics to the equation. If the cohort characteristics are good at accounting for the variability associated with cohorts, then the vari-ance associated with random effects of cohorts (u_k) will be reduced in this model. In the examples, and in Equations (5.1) and (5.2), we have used the cohort effects as the random effect, but it is possible to designate the period effect as the random effect or the age effect as the random effect.

In the APC ANOVA approach the variance is decomposed using the fact that the predicted value of y is an estimable function. Therefore, even though the individual age, period, and cohort coefficients are not estimable, given that the predicted value of y is estimable, the variance accounted for by the age, period, and cohort effects is estimable. Next, I describe why in the mixed model the age, period, and cohort effects are statistically identified. I begin with a simple analogous procedure.

Within the APC tradition there is general agreement that it is impossible to uniquely estimate the individual age, period, and cohort effects without placing a constraint on the model. However, the following two-step strategy provides estimates of age, period, and cohort effects: let cohort effects be represented by the residuals of an initial model in which age and period are considered fixed. Proceed by regressing the age–period-specific dependent variable on the age and period effect coded categorical variables. Then com-pute the residuals for the age–period cells as $(y_{ij} - \hat{y}_{ij})$. It would seem that the effects for cohorts are contained in these residuals, specifically on the cohort diagonals of the residuals placed in an age–period table. We could compute the mean of these residuals for each cohort diagonal. These would represent the random residuals associated with the cohort effects. If, for example, the fourth earliest cohort is particularly prone to mortality due to tuberculosis, its residuals should tend to be positive; if the eighth earliest cohort is rela-tively low in its propensity to tuberculosis mortality, its residuals should tend to be negative. Perhaps these cohort effects should be weighted, since they are based on different numbers of cases/cells. We might consider regression toward the mean based on the reliability of these estimates (based on the number of cases). Whatever is the best technical way of handling these resid-uals; however, they contain some useful information about the cohort effects.

There is, unfortunately, a fundamental problem with this approach, if it is intended to determine the age, period, and cohort effects. Entering the age and period effects in the first step gives them credit not only for the effects associated with these two factors, but also any linear effects due to cohorts. Note that even though this two-step model is identified, one will get different results for the age effects if one uses cohorts and periods as the fixed effects and determines the age effects based on the residuals. The effects of age differ systematically depending upon whether age is treated as a fixed or random effect.

Returning to the APCMM, it is identified for a similar reason. The standard model specifies that the residuals (ϵ_{ijk}) and the random effects (u_k) are independently identically distributed and, as Snijders (2005:665) notes, "the assumption is made that the random effects are uncorrelated with the explanatory variables." Thus, the random cohort effects are independent of the effects of period and age and, since these are completely confounded with the linear effects of cohort, they are independent of the linear effects of cohort. The results are similar to those for the APC ANOVA approach where the deviations of cohorts around their trend line are identified, although these random effects are not exactly the same as the deviations for the APC ANOVA approach.

A third way to consider why this model is identified is suggested by the matrix form of the linear mixed model:

$$y = X\beta + Zu + \epsilon. \tag{5.3}$$

where y is a column vector of observations on the dependent variable (the age–period-specific rates) and X is the design matrix for the fixed effects. For the APCMM when cohorts are treated as the random effect, X consists of a column of ones for the intercept, $I - 1$ columns for the effect coded age categorical variables, and $J - 1$ columns for the effect coded period categorical variables (if cohort characteristics are used, there is a column in the X matrix for each of them). There is one row for each of the age–period-specific observations. β is a vector of the fixed effect coefficients. The X-matrix should in general be invertible, since it consists of only two of the factors (in this case the age and period effect coded categorical variables). Z is the design matrix for the random effects, in this case the random cohort effects. It consists of a column for each of the cohorts and a row corresponding to each of the age–period-specific observations. If the age–period-specific observation in the row is an observation that is in the cohort represented by the column there is a 1 in that column and a 0 if not. The vector of random effects u is a column vector of the corresponding random effects with (in this case) one entry per cohort and ϵ is a column vector of residual errors with one row for each age–period-specific observation. In sum, the fixed effect regression for age and period is identified and the residuals due to cohorts are based on the residual variance in the dependent variable associated with the different cohorts.

To provide insights into the APCMM approach and to draw comparisons with the APC ANOVA approach, I again use the breast cancer data. The

TABLE 5.2

Random Variances in Mixed Models When Cohorts
or Periods or Ages Are Treated As the Random Variable

	Linear Mixed Model for Logged Rates		
	Random Variance	Chibar2(1)[a]	P <
Cohorts	0.0104	24.09	0.0001
Periods	0.0021	18.95	0.0001
Ages	0.4162	124.5	0.0001
	Poisson Mixed Model for Counts		
	Random Variance	Chibar2(1)[a]	P <
Cohorts	0.0834	123.62	0.0001
Periods	0.0339	37.33	0.0001
Ages	0.5791	4544.71	0.0001

[a] The Chibar2 statistic is based on the likelihood ratio chi-square of the fixed effects model compared to the model that contains both the fixed effects and the random effects, but the p-value takes into consideration that the variance will be positive.

findings in Table 5.2 are based on APCMMs that treat, in turn, cohorts as the random effect, periods as the random effect, and ages as the random effect. The results are summarized in terms of the random variance accounted for by cohorts, periods, and ages. In each case, the random variances for cohorts, ages, and periods are statistically significant. As with the tests for the unique variances associated with these variables using the APC ANOVA approach of Section 5.2, it is clear that the most important effect, in terms of the unique variance associated with it, after controlling for the other two factors is age. We once again would conclude that effects of age, period, and cohort account for a statistically significant amount of variance after taking the other two factors into account. This is the case both for the APCMM linear analysis and for the APCMM Poisson analysis.

Figure 5.1 shows the random effects of cohorts, ages, and periods when the other two factors are fixed effects in the linear APCMM. Given the earlier discussion, parts of these results are not surprising. The random effect solutions show no linear trend in the coefficient estimates (the slopes of these coefficients are zero in each case). Each of these figures also includes the deviations from linearity of the same factor based on the methods in Chapter 4 on estimable functions. These deviations are derived from any of the constrained estimates by calculating the linear trend for the coefficients for a factor and then the deviations of the coefficients from this trend. They are nearly identical to the random effects from the linear mixed models. These mixed model random effects nearly match the deviations from linear trends that are estimable functions. The APC ANOVA results are based on these estimable deviations.

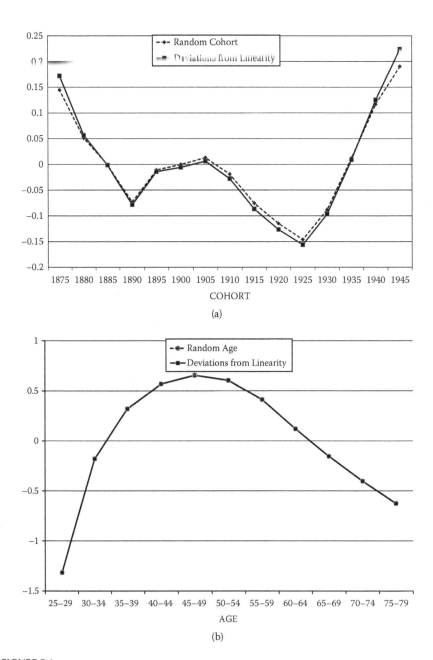

FIGURE 5.1
Random effects for the linear APCMM approach and deviations from linearity for the OLS regression model. (a) Random cohort effects and the cohort deviations from linearity. (b) Random age effects and the age deviations from linearity. (c) Random period effects and the period deviations from linearity. *(continued)*

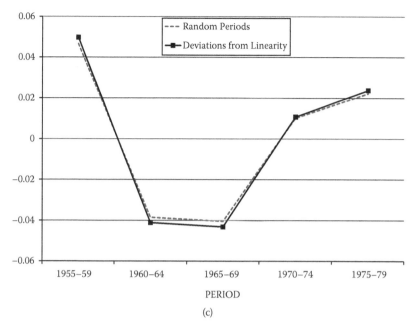

(c)

FIGURE 5.1 (continued).
Random effects for the linear APCMM approach and deviations from linearity for the OLS regression model. (a) Random cohort effects and the cohort deviations from linearity. (b) Random age effects and the age deviations from linearity. (c) Random period effects and the period deviations from linearity.

Even though the trends in the data-generating parameters are not known for these random effect coefficients, we can say some things about the data-generating parameters. If there were no trend, we could conclude that the trend in birth cohort rates is negative for the earliest cohorts and positive for the most recent cohorts. If a "strong negative trend" were added to Figure 5.1a, we could make it so that the trend was monotonic and negative for the cohort effects over time. This, however, would not change the following statement about the trend: the trend in birth cohort rates is more negative for the earlier cohorts than the more recent cohorts. The same statement holds if we make the trend positive. The trend is more negative (less positive) for the earlier cohorts than the latter cohorts. We know that this statement holds true for the data-generating parameters in the APC ANOVA case and are confident that it is nearly true in the APCMM situation. In a similar manner the deviations from linearity/random effects for the age and period can be interpreted. Note that for the age curve in Figure 5.1b, this interpretation fits with what is known of age and proneness to breast cancer mortality. The age trend in breast cancer mortality age is relatively more positive at the younger ages than at the older ages. This is what Figure 5.1b for the random effects of age shows, although substantively one would want to add a positive slope to these random effects.

Figure 5.2 displays the fixed effects from the linear APCMM and the fixed effects from an OLS regression model in which two of the factors are included as independent variables and the other factor is not included. The fixed effects for the APCMM and the fixed effects from an OLS regression model are strikingly similar for the situation in which cohort is the random variable (age and period fixed effects) in Figure 5.2a and when period is the random variable (age and cohort are the fixed effects) in Figure 5.2b; and they are mainly similar when the random effect is age (period and cohort are the fixed effects) in Figure 5.2c. In Figure 5.2c the fixed effects for cohorts from the APCMM analysis show a nearly linear decline in the breast cancer rate over time, whereas the results from the OLS analysis are more complex with a near leveling of the trend for the cohort effects from 1895 through 1910. However, the overall downward linear trends are similar.

More important, the choice of the factor to use as the random effect can greatly influence the estimates of the fixed effects. This is best seen in Figure 5.2 by comparing the fixed effects of cohort when period is the random variable (Figure 5.2b) and when age is the random variable (Figure 5.2c). When period is the random variable the cohort effects have a slight upward trend from the earliest to the most recent cohort while the cohort effects

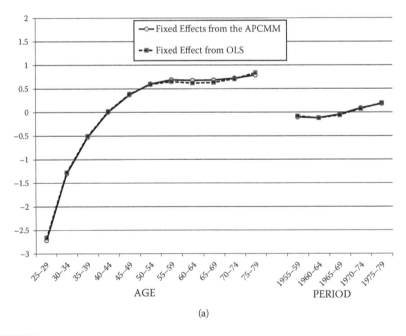

(a)

FIGURE 5.2
Fixed effects based on the linear APCMM and OLS regression model. (a) Cohort as the random effect. (b) Period as the random effect. (c) Age as the random effect. *(continued)*

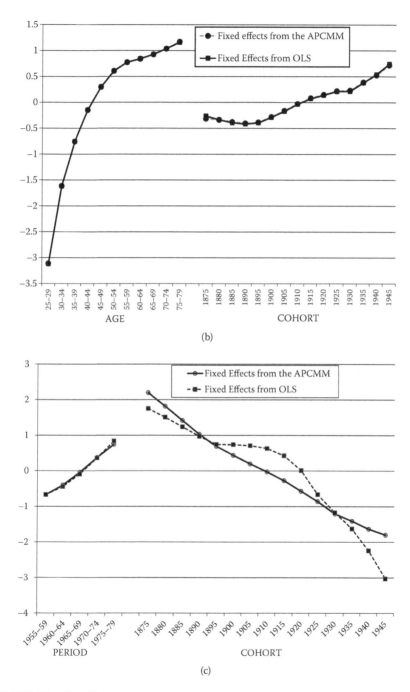

FIGURE 5.2 (continued).
Fixed effects based on the linear APCMM and OLS regression model. (a) Cohort as the random effect. (b) Period as the random effect. (c) Age as the random effect.

when age is the random variable show a marked downward trend. The decision concerning which variable should be treated as random in this simple mixed model has important ramifications for the results from the fixed effect portion of the analysis, and it is not necessarily clear which variable or variables should be considered fixed or random. Similar comments apply to the fixed effects from the OLS analysis that enters only two of the factors. Here, the trend in the factors depends on which two factors are entered into the equation and which one is left out of the analysis. Although one might quibble about which variable is the best to treat as a random effect and which two should be treated as fixed effects, we should not trust the fixed effect estimates or the random effect estimates unless there is some reason to suspect that effects associated with the factor classified as random do not trend with time for the parameters that generated the outcome data.

Turning to the Poisson APCMM regression, note that as reported in Table 5.2 each of the random effects from the Poisson APCMM analysis for breast cancer counts is statistically significant. For both the linear and Poisson APCMM, the unique variance associated with age is the greatest of any of the factors. We can see from Figure 5.3 that there is no linear trend in these random effects based on the Poisson analysis; when these effects are

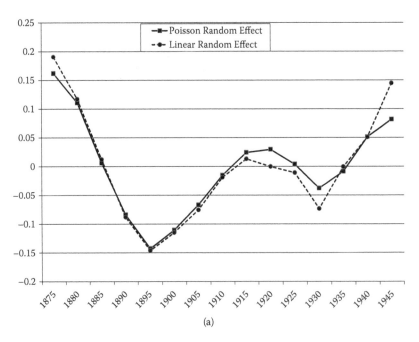

(a)

FIGURE 5.3
Random effects from the Poisson APCMM and the linear APCMM. (a) Random cohort effects. (b) Random age effects. (c) Random period effects. *(continued)*

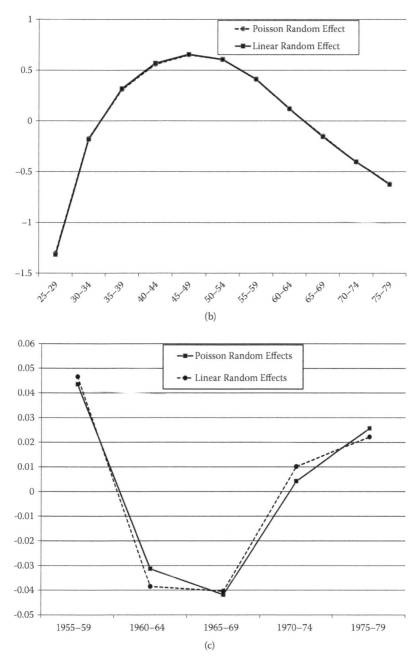

FIGURE 5.3 (continued).
Random effects from the Poisson APCMM and the linear APCMM. (a) Random cohort effects. (b) Random age effects. (c) Random period effects.

regressed on time the slopes are zero. This figure contains both the random effects based on the Poisson APCMM analyses and those based on the linear APCMM analyses. They are nearly identical when ages are the random effects (Figure 5.3b) and quite similar when cohorts and when period are treated as the random effects (Figures 5.3a and 5.3c). When the fixed effects from the Poisson APCMM were compared to the standard linear APCMM (though these results are not shown), the results are also quite similar. The fixed effects from the Poisson APCMM are nearly equivalent to those for the linear APCMM depicted in Figure 5.2. If one were to try to interpret the fixed effects from these analyses, note again that it matters which factor is treated as random. Since the random effects, by construction, have no linear trend, the two fixed effects take credit for any linear trend in the random effects that might be associated with the data-generating parameters.

As a brief summary for this section and an extension to more than a single random variable I note that the APCMM is identified without any additional constraints being added to the model. In the case of using only a single random factor the APCMM model constrains the results for the random factor to have no trend with time. The two factors that are treated as fixed effects take credit for their own effects and any linear effects associated with the random factor. In this case, the random effects are nearly equivalent to the deviations from linear trends described in Chapter 4, and those deviations are estimable. The analyst is on solid ground, as long as these random effects are interpreted as the deviations of these effects from linear trends. Tests for the significance of these random effects can also be seen as tests for the nonlinear effects of the random factor. If the random effects are statistically significant then the random factor significantly improves the fit of the model even without being given any credit for linear effects.

This is a sufficient test for the effects of the random factor in that if this test is statistically significant then the random factor is associated with a statistically significant amount of variance in the outcome variable. This, however, is not a necessary condition. Even if the random variance is not statistically significant for the factor, if the factor being treated as random were given credit for any linear trend that it has, it might account for a statistically significant amount of variance in the outcome variable. The individual effect coefficients in the fixed effects portion of the models should not be interpreted as estimates of the parameters that generated the outcome values. These coefficients are confounded with whatever linear trends might be associated with the random factor. For the fixed effects, this is quite similar to (though not exactly the same) as a regression model in which only two of the factors are included in the regression.

The statistical identification status of the APCMM does not depend upon having two of the factors as fixed effects and one of them treated as random. Models can be analyzed in which two of the factors are random and even models in which all three of the factors are random (that is, there are no fixed effects). For these models the random factors are specified as crossed (Yang and Land 2006), since they are not nested one within the other. If age and period are random, then each of the age–period-specific rates or counts is in a particular period, but that period is not nested within a particular age, but instead is crossed with the age factor. Similarly, if the age and cohort factors are random, the age and cohort factors are crossed. Each of these models is identified without any additional explicit constraint. In these models it is not atypical for the random effects to show some trend, but that trend is different from when the factor is treated as a fixed effect. It is clear that such models do not solve the problem of how to distribute the trends so that the effect coefficients provide unbiased or nearly unbiased estimates of the data-generating parameters.

5.4 Hierarchical APC Model

This book focuses on APC models that use aggregate-level data of the kind found in many sources of "official statistics." There is, however, a technique developed by Yang and Land (2006) that focuses on "aggregate" or "macrolevel" data for periods and cohorts, and treats age as an individual-level variable. To use this approach one must have individual-level data such as that available from repeated cross-sectional surveys; for example, data from the General Social Survey or self-reported health from the National Health Interview Survey. Yang and Land suggest analyzing this data using hierarchical modeling with age at the individual level (level 1) and period and cohort at the macrolevel (level 2). They label their approach the hierarchical age–period–cohort (HAPC) model, and they use a cross-classified random effects model (CCREM) for the crossed (rather than nested) period and cohort random effects. That is, they use an HAPC CCREM approach to modeling age, period, and cohort effects.

More formally, using the notation of hierarchical models (Yang 2011), the level 1 or within-cell model can be written as

$$Y_{ijk} = \beta_{0jk} + \beta_1 X_{1ijk} + \beta_2 X_{2ijk} + \ldots + \beta_P X_{Pijk} + e_{ijk},$$ (5.4)

where $i = 1, 2, \ldots, n_{jk}$ for the individuals within period j and cohort k; $j = 1, \ldots, J$ periods and $k = 1, \ldots, K$ birth cohorts, and the residuals (e_{ijk}) are normally distributed with a mean of zero and variance equals σ^2. The continuous explanatory variables (often most of the X variables) are grand mean centered. In the simplest and most commonly employed HAPC analysis, the researcher does not attempt to model influences other than the period and cohort effects at level ? Then the level 2 or between-cell model is written as

$$\beta_{0jk} = \gamma_0 + u_{0j} + v_{0k},$$ (5.5)

where the period random effects (u_{0j}) are normally distributed with a mean of zero and variance τ_u, and the cohort random effects (v_{0k}) are normally distributed with a mean of zero and a variance of τ_v. Equation (5.5) models the intercept in Equation (5.4) by making the cell mean go up or down depending upon the effects of the level 2 random variables of periods (u_{0j}) and cohorts (v_{0k}). The combined or mixed-effects model can then be written as

$$Y_{ijk} = \gamma_0 + \beta_1 X_{1ijk} + \beta_2 X_{2ijk} + \ldots + \beta_P X_{Pijk} + u_{0j} + v_{0k} + e_{ijk}.$$ (5.6)

Here, γ_0 is the expected value when all of the level 1 variables are at zero, u_{0j} is the residual random effect of period j (the contribution of period j averaged over all cohorts), and v_{0k} is the residual random effect of cohort k (the contribution of cohort k averaged over all periods). One of the advantages of this model is that other predictor variables (in addition to age) can be used to predict the effects of individual characteristics on the dependent variable; for example, we can have X variables for age, age squared, education, gender, marital status, and so on.

Yang and associates (2006, 2011, 2013) know that this model is identified, but there seems to have been some confusion at different times concerning why it is identified. In their initial presentation of the HAPC model, they placed special emphasis on adding an age-squared component to the level 1 model: "In the case of the substantive analysis described here, this application is facilitated by the specification of a nonlinear parametric form for one of the age, period, or cohort dimensions that breaks the under-identification problem of the classical APC accounting model" (Yang and Land 2006:92). Until it is shown how this strategy solves the identification problem, researchers should remain skeptical that this quadratic component somehow solves the underidentification problem. Adding a squared age variable to the fixed effect portion of the model that contains the age variable should not affect any potential linear dependency between age, period, and cohort.

The second factor mentioned by Yang and associates as identifying the model involves using unequal age, period, and cohort intervals: "Note that individual-level data available in survey designs allow age intervals to differ from period intervals. Unequal age, period, and cohort intervals then break the exact linear dependency of the three variables in the APC accounting model suited for aggregate population-level data" (Zheng, Yang, and Land 2011:960). This inequality of intervals certainly can be used to identify the APC model. This approach, however, is available for individual- or aggregate-level data where unequal intervals can almost always be constructed. Osmond and Gardner (1989) note that this does not resolve the identification problem without introducing a constraint. Different groupings produce different constraints and produce different results.* Zheng, Yang, and Land (2011:960) are aware of this problem noting, "Results may be sensitive to the choice of interval widths, because longer widths may allow a higher degree of over-identification." Despite this caution, they and others who use the HAPC approach use unequal age and/or period and/or cohort intervals even though the results will shift depending upon the intervals used (Luo and Hodges 2013).

Yang and Land (2013:191) mention a third factor: "The HAPC framework does not incur the identification problem because the three effects are not assumed to be linear and additive at the same level of analysis." This is what I find for the APCMM model. The analogy of first finding fixed effects for two of the factors and then using residuals to find the effects of the third factor from earlier in this chapter is close to this conception. More exact is the matrix depiction of the mixed/hierarchical model in which the fixed effects appear in the X-matrix and the random effects appear in the Z-matrix (Equation 5.3). That is, the three effects are not assumed to be linear and additive at the same level of analysis.

Yang and Land's (2006, 2013) model is very similar to the APCMM presented in the previous section except that the APCMM uses only aggregate-level data. The APCMM can be formulated with age at level 1 and the cross-classified random effects for periods and cohorts at level 2. The model is identified whether the effect-coded version of age is used as the level 1 variable or a continuously measured age variable is used as in the HAPC model. This model runs with no quadratic age component and without overlapping categorization of the age and/or period and/or cohort factors. It can also be run, as illustrated in the examples of this chapter, with a single one of the factors as random. In that sense the APCMM like the HAPC "does not incur the identification problem." The APCMM might be viewed as a solution to the long-standing problem of identification in aggregate-level APC analysis described in this book.

Unfortunately, the APCMM does not solve the APC identification problem in terms of providing unbiased estimates of the parameters that generated the outcome values of the dependent variable. One reason for this conclusion can be seen in Figure 5.2, where it is obvious that the factor that is chosen as the random factor greatly affects the estimates of the two fixed-effect

---

* For example, using the APC constrained models of Chapter 2, if the researcher normally would use 5-year periods, 5-year cohorts, and 5-year age groups she could decide to construct 10-year cohort groupings. If there were ten 5-year cohorts, this would impose the following five constraints: coh1 = coh2, coh3 = coh4, …, coh9 = coh10. Periods and age groups could then take on different values within cohorts breaking the linear dependency between ages, periods, and cohorts. This identifies the model in the traditional APC aggregate-level situation. But different constraints will produce different results. This is also the case for the HAPC model. Typically, more than a single constraint is produced by using such unequal intervals.

factors. This is similar to the conclusions drawn in O'Brien, Hudson, and Stockard (2008). Specifying two fixed effects as additive at one level and the third effect random, or one effect fixed and two random allows the model to be statistically identified, but it does not result in a plausible division of the linear trends in the age effects, period effects, and cohort effects to each of these factors. This division systematically depends upon which variables are treated as random and which are treated as fixed (its own constraint on how the linear components are apportioned). This conclusion extends to the HAPC model.

5.5 Empirical Example Using Homicide Offending Data

5.5.1 Applying the APC ANOVA Approach

To illustrate the ANOVA and APCMM approaches, I use age–period-specific homicide arrests data for the United States from the Federal Bureau of Investigation (various years). That data appears in Table 5.3 with the age–period-specific arrest rates per 100,000 residents listed first and the age–period-specific number of homicide arrests listed second (in parentheses) for each of the 5-year age groups (15–19 to 60–64) in each of the periods 1965 to 2010. To conduct the Poisson analyses, we also need to know the number of people in each of the age–period-specific groups. For these data we can calculate the number of people in each age–period-specific group as the number of arrests in each age–period-specific group times 100,000 and then divided by the age–period-specific rate per 100,000.

This data is supplemented with two characteristics of the cohorts. Relative cohort size (RCS) is measured when the members of the birth cohort are 15–19 years of age. It is the percentage of the United States resident population aged 15–64 who are 15–19 when the birth cohort members are 15–19 years of age. The U.S. Census Bureau (various years) provides the data for these calculations. RCS measures the cohort's percentage of the population that stretches from their birth cohort and into the parental generation. This measure of RCS has been used in part because it measures baby boom, baby bust, and normal cohorts, and does so at a crucial life stage for the cohort (O'Brien, Stockard, and Isaacson 1999). Baby boom cohorts tend to have fewer adults per child, larger class sizes in schools, fewer entry level jobs per entry level job seeker when the cohort enters the job market, and other disadvantages. The other cohort characteristic is the percentage of the birth cohort born to nonmarried mothers. Annual percentages were drawn from two sources: U.S. Bureau of the Census (1946, 1990) and Martin, Hamilton, Ventura et al. (2012). For the cohort born between 1940 and 1944, for example, I averaged the annual percentages of live births that were to nonmarried mothers.

TABLE 5.3

Age–Period-Specific Homicide Offending Arrest Data per 100,000 and the Age–Period-Specific Number of Arrests (in Parentheses) for the United States: Ages 15–19 to 60–64 from 1965 to 2010

Ages	Periods									
	1965	1970	1975	1980	1985	1990	1995	2000	2005	2010
15–19	9.07	17.22	17.54	18.00	16.32	35.17	35.08	14.63	13.87	10.89
	(1536)	(3311)	(3723)	(3799)	(3028)	(6245)	(6372)	(3017)	(2918)	(2371)
20–24	15.18	23.75	25.62	23.97	21.10	29.10	31.93	18.46	18.70	13.08
	(2035)	(3938)	(4949)	(5124)	(4432)	(5567)	(5790)	(3740)	(3933)	(2848)
25–29	14.69	20.09	21.05	18.88	16.79	18.00	16.76	10.90	11.85	8.63
	(1650)	(2733)	(3617)	(3719)	(3652)	(3820)	(3187)	(2084)	(2378)	(1848)
30–34	11.70	16.00	15.81	15.23	12.58	12.44	10.05	6.63	6.80	5.94
	(1292)	(1841)	(2234)	(2704)	(2550)	(2726)	(2200)	(1280)	(1366)	(1212)
35–39	9.76	13.13	12.83	12.32	9.60	9.38	7.25	5.41	4.69	4.10
	(1166)	(1454)	(1486)	(1734)	(1700)	(1874)	(1619)	(1111)	(986)	(831)
40–44	7.41	10.10	10.52	8.80	7.50	6.81	5.47	3.74	3.69	2.88
	(918)	(1208)	(1176)	(1032)	(1054)	(1212)	(1109)	(848)	(843)	(606)
45–49	5.56	7.50	7.32	6.76	5.31	5.17	3.67	2.30	3.09	2.39
	(632)	(911)	(862)	(747)	(619)	(714)	(641)	(518)	(696)	(540)
50–54	4.60	5.68	4.91	4.36	4.32	3.38	2.68	1.70	1.74	1.71
	(481)	(634)	(588)	(510)	(473)	(384)	(366)	(344)	(347)	(377)
55–59	3.13	4.38	3.34	3.28	3.31	2.36	2.50	0.89	1.22	1.19
	(297)	(439)	(356)	(381)	(375)	(247)	(277)	(158)	(211)	(233)
60–64	2.38	2.78	2.99	2.16	1.90	1.77	1.39	0.64	0.76	0.73
	(180)	(241)	(281)	(219)	(209)	(188)	(139)	(87)	(99)	(123)

Source: Data from Federal Bureau of Investigation, various years, *Crime in the United States,* Washington D.C.: Government Printing Office.

O'Brien, Stockard, and Isaacson (1999) note that such cohorts are more likely to have children that grow up in poverty, live in poor neighborhoods, have poorer access to medical care, are less likely to have adequate monitoring and supervision, and are otherwise disadvantaged (see O'Brien et al. 1999, for more details and citations).

The values of these two cohort characteristics are the same for members of a birth cohort no matter what their age or the particular period. An advantage of these measures is that they are not linearly dependent on age and period, and so do not create identification problems. A disadvantage is that they are likely not to capture the full association between the dependent variable (age–period-specific homicide offending rates) and cohort membership after controlling for age and period. To the extent that this is the case they will underestimate the importance of cohorts and produce biased estimates of the age and period effects. These models are covered in depth in Chapter 6 that features factor-characteristic models. In the present analysis, these characteristics are used to assess how much of the variance in age–period-specific homicide rates, which is uniquely associated with cohorts, can be accounted for by these cohort characteristics.

The ANOVA approach for partitioning variance is used first. It determines whether the evidence is sufficient to conclude that age, period, and cohort each account for a unique portion of the logged age–period-specific variability in the rates of homicide offending. Table 5.4 provides the answer to this question. Using an OLS regression analysis approach, we find that in each case the unique variance accounted for by each of these factors is statistically significant at the .0001 level. Cohorts add 3.1% to the variance accounted for by the logged age–period-specific homicide offending rates accounted for by a model that includes only the age and period factors. Periods add 6.1% to the variance accounted for by a model that includes the age and cohort factors. Ages add 3.3% to the variance accounted for by a model that includes the period and cohort factors. Comparing the unique variance accounted for may not be the best way to compare these factors, because the different factors do not all have the same number of parameters used to account for additional variance (17 for cohorts and 8 each for periods and ages). In terms of the adjusted R^2, the additional adjusted variances accounted for are 3.2% cohorts, 7.9% for periods, and 4.3% for ages.

Using Poisson regression to analyze these data, the second panel in Table 5.4 indicates that in terms of the significance of the improvement of

TABLE 5.4

Tests for the Unique Effects of Cohorts, Periods, and Ages after Controlling for the Other Two Factors for the Homicide Offense Data

| | OLS Regression of Logged Rates | | | |
	Degrees of Freedom	P <	F	$R^2_{increment}$
Cohorts	F(17, 64)	0.0001	7.06	0.031
Periods	F(8,64)	0.0001	29.13	0.061
Ages	F(8,64)	0.0001	16.28	0.033

| | Poisson Regression of Counts | | |
	Degrees of Freedom	P <	Chibar2[a]
Cohorts	Chi2(17)	0.0001	5366.94
Periods	Chi2(8)	0.0001	9857.84
Ages	Chi2(8)	0.0001	5899.16

[a] The Chibar2 statistic is based on the likelihood ratio chi-square of the fixed effects model compared to the model that contains both the fixed effects and the random effects, but the p-value takes into consideration that the variance will be positive.

fit associated with each of these factors each factor is important. These chi-square values are based on the improvement in the fit of the model when we add the final factor to a model that includes the other two.

For the homicide offense data, two cohort characteristics are used: relative cohort size (RCS) and the percentage of nonmarital births (NMB). These cohort characteristics are logged and used in place of the cohort factor. Two advantages are that the model is identified and that two mechanisms are specified that might produce the variance associated with cohorts. Both of these cohort characteristics are statistically significant and positively associated with the logged age–period-specific homicide offending rates after controlling for the age and period effects in both the OLS and Poisson regression analyses. These characteristics are associated with a greater tendency for the members of specific cohorts to commit homicide across the years covered by these data as hypothesized in O'Brien, Stockard, and Isaacson (1999).

Focusing on variance accounted for by the three different factors, cohorts uniquely account for 3.08% of the variance in homicide offending (in the OLS results reported in Table 5.4). This is based on the R^2 for the full model (0.9836) minus the R^2 for the model without the cohort categorical variables (0.9528). When the cohort characteristics are used, along with the age and period factors to predict the logged age–period-specific homicide rates, then $R^2 = 0.9797$. The model that contains age effects, period effects, and the cohort characteristics adds 0.0269 (= .9797 − .9528) to the proportion of the variance accounted for in a model that contains only age and period effects. The two cohort characteristics account for 87% of the variance uniquely associated with cohorts [= (0.0269/0.0308) × 100].

Criminologists are particularly interested in the effects of cohorts when it comes to examining the age distribution of homicide offending, because there has been some controversy surrounding this age distribution. Hirschi and Gottfredson (1983) have called this relationship invariant: invariant not in the absolute rates, but in terms of the proportion of the cases in the different age groups. This distribution was indeed remarkably stable in the United States until the late 1980s when what was labeled as the epidemic of youth homicide occurred. This epidemic can be seen in the data of Table 5.3, which shows the homicide rate for different age groups over time from 1965 through 2010. From 1985 to 1990 the rate of homicide offending for those 15–19 increase by 116%, the rates for those 20–24 increased by 38%, and the rates for those aged 30–34 to 60–64 all decreased. In 1995 these rates remained at similar levels while the rates for those 25–29 to 60–64 all decreased (with the exception of the rates for those 55–59).

We can check if these were statistically significant shifts in the age distributions across periods by introducing interactions to account for this upturn in youth violence. The four interaction terms introduced are for the youngest two age groups in the years 1990 and 1995: age(15–19) × period1990, age(15–19) × period1995, age(20–24) × period1990, and age(20–24) × period1995. When these four interactions are added to the full model that contains the age, period, and cohort factors with a single constraint, they account for a statistically significant amount of variance [$F_{(4, 60)} = 2.76$, $p < .01$]. Note that these four interactions can be entered into the model, because these interactions are not linearly related to the age, period, and cohort factors. They are estimable functions that are deviations from linearity and do not depend on the constraint used. When they are added to the model that contains the age and period factors and the two cohort characteristics, they account for an additional amount of variance in this model also [$F(4, 69) = 3.75$, $p < .01$)].

Some researchers may object that if age and period factors account for 95.28% of the variance in the age–period-specific rates of homicide offending, then the amount of additional variance accounted for by cohorts (3.08%) is trivial. The graphs presented in Figure 5.4 are designed to show the importance of these cohort effects. These cohort effects appear to be responsible for a major portion of the epidemic of youth homicide that so fascinated and alarmed criminologists. Such substantively important phenomena can get lost by concentrating on R^2 in a regression analysis. Two major factors in determining the rates of homicide offending are age and period (others are gender and race). The overall rate of homicides during the years covered in these analyses differed by a ratio of nearly 2 to 1. The age variation is seen in the graphs in Figure 5.4; it is not uncommon for the highest and lowest rates in this age range (15–19 to 60–64) to differ by a ratio exceeding 6 to 1. These two factors account for over 95% of the variance (note they take credit for any linear trend in the cohort effects), but within each graph we see important distinctions between predictions that include and exclude cohorts.

Up until 1985 homicide offending followed a stable pattern with those in the 20–24 age category exhibiting the highest rates; then the "epidemic of youth homicide" occurred. This is evident in Figure 5.4b and in Figure 5.4c where the rates for those age 15–19 were the highest; by the year 2000 (Figure 5.4d) the highest rates were again for the 20–24 age group. During the peak of the epidemic of youth homicide in 1990, using the model with cohorts for prediction accounted for 35% of the gap between the observed logged rate of homicide offending for those 15–19 and that predicted without cohorts in the model. In 1995 cohorts accounted for 46% of that gap. After the peak of offending returned to the age group 20–24 in 2000, cohorts accounted for 66% of the gap between the age–period predicted rate and the observed rate. Although graphs based on Poisson regression are not presented, they are quite similar.

I conclude that cohorts are important for understanding changes in the age distribution of homicide offending over time. Cohorts contribute uniquely to the variance accounted for in the age–period-specific rates of homicide offending, and this unique variance accounted for is an estimable function when using the APC ANOVA approach. It is an unbiased estimate of the unique variance accounted for by cohorts for the generating parameters. The graphs in Figure 5.4 show that these cohort effects are substantively important.

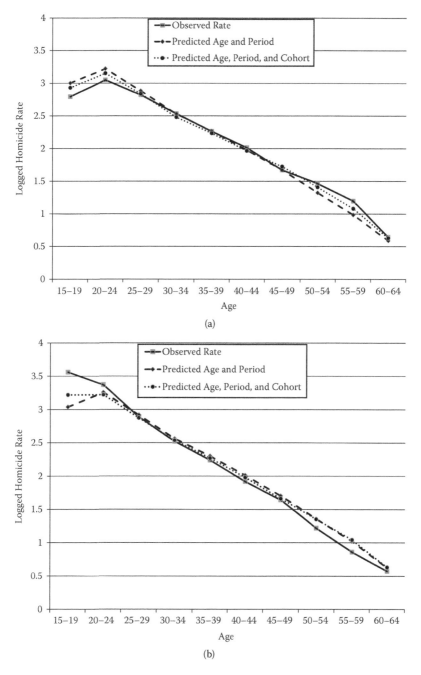

(a)

(b)

FIGURE 5.4
Logged rates of homicide offending and predictions based on age and period factors and age, period, and cohort factors. (a) Homicide offending 1985. (b) Homicide offending 1990. (c) Homicide offending 1995. (d) Homicide offending 2000. *(continued)*

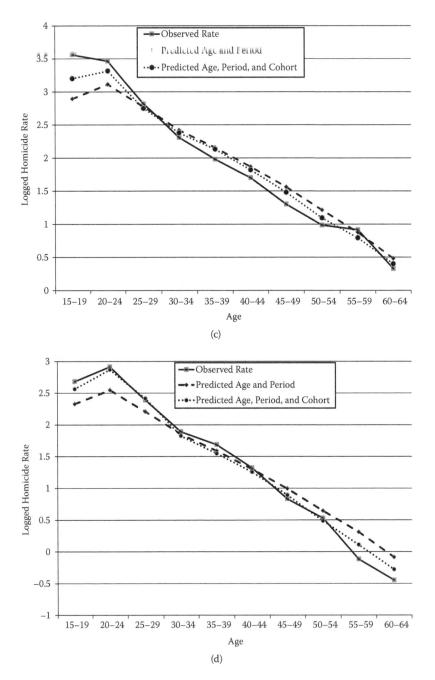

FIGURE 5.4 (continued).

Logged rates of homicide offending and predictions based on age and period factors and age, period, and cohort factors. (a) Homicide offending 1985. (b) Homicide offending 1990. (c) Homicide offending 1995. (d) Homicide offending 2000.

5.5.2 Applying the APCMM Approach

In this section the mixed-model approach is implemented to estimate the variance associated with the random cohort effects, the random period effects, and the random age effects. These analyses are conducted for both the APCMM linear model approach using the logged rates of homicide offending and with the APCMM Poisson model approach using the age–period-specific counts of homicide offending and "exposure" based on the number of U.S. residents in the particular age–period-specific category. These results appear in Table 5.5. These random effects are all statistically significant at the .0001 level for cohorts, ages, and periods for both the linear and Poisson models. In both cases periods seem to account for the most variance of any of the random components (0.0764) in the linear APCMM approach and (0.1035) in the Poisson APCMM approach, but for the Poisson analysis cohorts are the second most important (0.0843) and ages are the least important (0.0385), while for the linear model ages are the second most important in terms of variance and cohorts are the least important. Note again, however, that the cohort random effects use more parameters than the age and period random effects. We do not expect the two analyses to be exactly the same, since one measures the variance of logged age–period-specific homicide offending rates and the other the variance of the logged age–period-specific counts of homicide offending (taking into consideration different population sizes for the age–period-specific groups).

TABLE 5.5

Random Variances in Mixed Models When Cohorts or Periods or Ages Are Treated As the Random Variable for the Age–Period-Specific Homicide Rates

	Linear Mixed Model with Homicide Rates		
	Random Variance	**Chibar2(1)[a]**	**P <**
Cohorts	0.0392	28.53	0.0001
Periods	0.0764	74.18	0.0001
Ages	0.0416	48.23	0.0001
	Poisson Mixed Model with Homicide Counts		
	Random Variance	**Chibar2(1)[a]**	**P <**
Cohorts	0.0843	5374.64	0.0001
Periods	0.1035	10618.60	0.0001
Ages	0.0385	6147.46	0.0001

[a] The Chibar2 statistic is based on the likelihood ratio chi-square of the fixed effects model compared to the model that contains both the fixed effects and the random effects, but the p-value takes into consideration that the variance will be positive.

The random effects on which these variances are based are depicted in Figure 5.5. This set of three graphs shows the random effects for both the linear APCMM and Poisson APCMM models for cohorts, ages, and periods. In each case, the random effects have no trend with time. Any linear components associated with these effects have been accounted for by the other two factors in the analysis. Thus, when interpreting the variance (.0843) associated with cohorts for the Poisson APCMM model with age and period fixed, this variance includes only the variance associated with the detrended effect of cohorts. The cohort effects before being detrended may be much larger. Just as important, when interpreting the fixed effects portion of this analysis the age and period coefficients take credit for any linear trend in cohorts. Note that we have not examined fixed effects from these analyses of homicide arrest data, in large part, because they are confounded with linear effects of the factor designated as the random effects factor.

These detrended random effects tell us something about the changes in the trends of these factors. For example, even if we add a positive or negative trend to the random period effects in Figure 5.5c, the earliest periods will show (in general) a relatively more positive/less negative trend in homicide offending than the most recent periods. For cohorts (Figure 5.5a) we can make the opposite statement that (in general) the earlier cohorts have a less

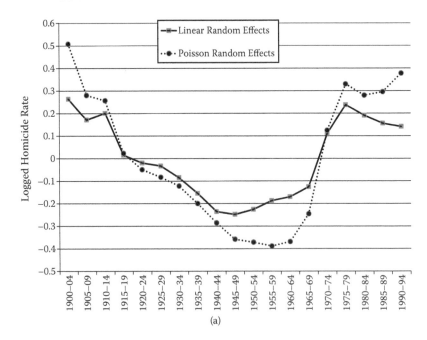

(a)

FIGURE 5.5
Random effects from linear APCMM and Poisson APCMM for homicide offending. (a) Random cohort effects. (b) Random age effects. (c) Random period effects. *(continued)*

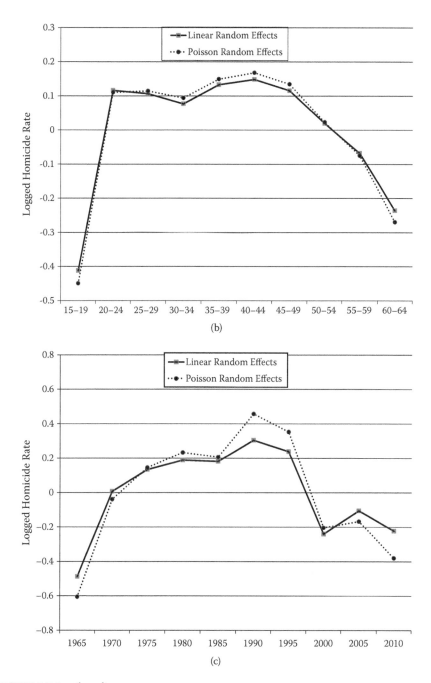

FIGURE 5.5 (continued).
Random effects from linear APCMM and Poisson APCMM for homicide offending. (a) Random cohort effects. (b) Random age effects. (c) Random period effects.

positive trend in homicide offending than the more recent cohorts. Although we could plot the fixed effects from the APCMM analyses they would tell us little of substantive interest, since they contain any linear trends that might be associated with the random effects and these effects differ depending upon which of the variables is chosen to be the random effects variable.

The APC ANOVA approach is able to determine the proportion of variance that is uniquely associated with cohorts that can be accounted for by the two cohort characteristics: the logged RCS and NMB. To determine this, we calculate $[(R^2_{apcc} - R^2_{ap}) / (R^2_{apc} - R^2_{ap})] \times 100$. The notation in the subscripts is *apcc* for a model with age, period, and cohort characteristics; *ap* for a model with age and period factors; and *apc* for a model with age, period, and cohort factors (with a single just identifying constraint).

To accomplish the same sort of partitioning with the APCMM for cohorts (as an example), we specify cohorts as the random effect with age and period as fixed effects and the output reports the random variance associated with cohorts. This is the amount of variance that is unique to cohorts. Then we add the logged values of RCS and NMB to the model as fixed effects, and the random variance estimated for this model is the variance associated with the random effects of cohorts that are not associated with the cohort characteristics. The proportion of the random variance in cohorts that is accounted for by the cohort characteristics can be calculated as

$$ 1 - \left[\frac{v_{0k:cc}}{v_{0k}} \right], $$

where v_{0k} is the random variance for cohorts in a model where ages and periods are the fixed effects and $v_{0k:cc}$ is the random variance for cohorts in a model in which ages, periods, and cohort characteristics are the fixed effects.

When these models are run with the age–period-specific homicide count data and the Poisson model is used, the random variance associated with cohorts is .0843 when we use age and periods as fixed effects. When the cohort characteristics are added to the fixed effects, the random variance associated with cohorts is reduced to .0066. The proportion of the random variance uniquely associated with cohorts in the Poisson regression that is accounted for by the two cohort characteristics is 92.17% [= 1 − (.0066/.0843)].

5.6 Conclusions

Variance partitioning, whether accomplished through the APC ANOVA approach or through the APCMM approach, leaves many questions unresolved. At the same time it answers some important questions about the effects of age, period, and cohort. This chapter shows that it is possible to determine that there are significant cohort effects and/or period effects and/or age effects, and this determination does not depend upon the constraint used. These tests provide evidence that the effects of the parameters that generated the outcome variable have a significant effect on the outcome values, because the deviations of the effects from their linear trend are estimable in the APC ANOVA case and "nearly so," though not technically so, in the APCMM situation. To justify this statement, note that the APCMM assessment of the random effects is for effects that show no trend over time.

On the other hand, it is not possible to show that there is not a significant amount of variance associated with any one of these factors. This is because any linear trend associated with a factor is not estimable or even "nearly so." A factor could show no deviations from linearity and, thus, not be associated with any of the variance in the dependent variable after the other two factors are entered into the equation. But for the parameters that generated the outcome variable, this factor may well have a substantial linear trend and would account for a statistically significant amount of variance in the outcome variable. The tests for unique variance for both the APC ANOVA approach and for the APCMM approach are not necessary and sufficient tests for whether a factor accounts for variance in the dependent variable.

Even though the underlying linear trends of the deviations from linearity for the random effects are not known, they tell us something about the relative trends within the factor under consideration If the cohort random effects in the APCMM analysis from the earliest cohort move downward and then at the middle cohort begin to move upward until the most recent cohort, we know that no matter what the linear trend for that factor might be (in terms of the generating parameters), the slope for the first set of cohorts is less positive than that for the second set of cohorts. The slope for the second set of cohorts might be negative, but the slope for the first set of cohorts will be more negative. We can learn something about the relative trends within a factor from these deviations that are themselves detrended.

As a general rule, I would advise against interpreting the fixed effects from either the OLS regression or the Poisson regression analysis that includes just two of the factors. For much the same reasons, I would also advise against interpreting the fixed effects when using linear APCMM or Poisson APCMM analyses. These analyses attribute any trend in the third factor (the one not in the regression or the one that is a random effect) to the two fixed effect factors. As noted in this chapter, these fixed effects can change radically depending on which factor is left out of the regression analysis or serves as a random variable.

The APCMM model runs without constraints, but in the solution for this model with one random factor and two fixed effect factors, the random effects are trendless.* Given this constraint, we would not claim that the

---

* This is the same kind of constraint introduced in Chapter 2, the zero linear trend (ZLT) constraint that identifies the APC model.

random effects or the coefficients associated with the other two factors are unbiased estimates of the data-generating parameters. That is not the case unless the true generating parameters happen to have no linear trend for the factor that the researcher designates as the random effect. The APCMM also runs without constraints for models in which two or three of the APC factors are treated as random effects. This solves the *statistical identification problem* in that the models run and they are statistically identified. The problem with these models as solutions to the APC identification problem is that they provide no assurance that the estimates they produce are suitable estimates of the parameters that generated the outcome values of the dependent variable. Stephen Fienberg notes in a recent comment on APC models in *Demography* (2013): "Thus, I simply note that when one changes a model via random effects … without strong prior information, one is still changing the model by fiat."

References

Clayton, D., and Schifflers, E. 1987. Models for temporal variation in cancer rates II: Age-period-cohort models. *Statistics in Medicine* 6:469–81.

Federal Bureau of Investigation. Various years. *Crime in the United States*. Washington D.C.: Government Printing Office.

Fienberg, S.E. 2013. Some personal history with APC analysis. *Demography*, 50:1981–85.

Hirschi, T., and M. Gottfredson. 1983. Age and the explanation of crime. *American Journal of Sociology* 3:552–84.

Luo, L., and J. Hodges. 2013. The cross-classified age-period-cohort model as a constrained estimator. Presented at the annual meeting of the Population Association of America, April.

Martin, J.A., B.E. Hamilton, and S.J. Ventura, et al. 2012. Births: Final data for 2010. *National Vital Statistics Reports*, vol. 61, no, 1. Hyattsville, MD: National Center for Health Statistics.

O'Brien, R.M., K. Hudson, and J. Stockard. 2008. A mixed model estimation of age, period, and cohort effects. *Sociological Methods & Research* 36:302–28.

O'Brien, R.M., and J. Stockard. 2009. Can cohort replacement explain changes in the relationship between age and homicide offending? *Journal of Quantitative Criminology* 25:79–101.

O'Brien, R.M., J. Stockard, and L. Isaacson. 1999. The enduring effects of cohort characteristics on age-specific homicide rates: 1960–1995. *American Journal of Sociology* 104:1061–95.

Osmond, C., and M.J. Gardner. 1989. Age, period, and cohort models: Non-overlapping cohorts don't resolve the identification problem. *American Journal of Epidemiology* 129:31–35.

Snijders, T.A.B. 2005. Fixed and random effects. In *Encyclopedia of Statistics in Behavioral Science*, vol. 2, eds. B.S. Everitt and D.C. Howell, 664–5. Chichester: Wiley.

StataCorp. 2013. *Stata Statistical Software: Release 13*. College Station, TX: StataCorp LP.

U.S. Bureau of the Census. Various years. Numbers 98, 114, 170, 519, 870, 1000, 1022, 1058, 1127, and for 1995-2010 online. *Current Population Surveys: Series P-25.* Washington D.C.: Government Printing Office.

U.S. Bureau of the Census. 1946, 1990. *Vital Statistics of the United States: Natality.* Washington D.C.: Government Printing Office.

Yang, Y. 2011. Aging, cohorts, and methods. In *Handbook of Aging and the Social Sciences* (7th edition), eds. R. Binstock and L.K. George, 17–30. San Diego: Academic Press.

Yang, Y., and K.C. Land. 2006. A mixed models approach to the age-period-cohort analysis of repeated cross-section surveys, with applications to data on trends in verbal test scores. *Sociological Methodology* 36:75–97.

Yang, Y., and K.C. Land. 2013. *Age-Period-Cohort Analysis: New Models, Methods, and Empirical Applications.* New York: Chapman & Hall.

Zheng, H., Y. Yang, and K.C. Land. 2011. Variance function regression in hierarchical age-period-cohort models: Applications to the study of self-reported health. *American Sociological Review* 76:955–83.

6

Factor-Characteristic Approach

> It is extremely important to keep in mind, however, that these models [factor-characteristic models] are not true APC models (although they are sometimes represented as such) and in no sense provide a solution to the age-period-cohort conundrum.
>
> **N.D. Glenn (2005:21)**

6.1 Introduction

The last chapter showed how to assess the variance uniquely associated with ages, periods, and cohorts, even though it is not possible to estimate the age, period, and cohort coefficients uniquely. It also strongly recommended not taking the fixed effects in such models as unbiased estimates of the parameters that generated the outcome values. These conclusions hold for APC ANOVA (age–period–cohort analysis of variance) and APCMM (age–period–cohort mixed model) approaches and extend to other hierarchical/mixed-model approaches.

In this chapter a different strategy is used to attempt to estimate the effects of age, period, and cohort. This strategy breaks the linear dependency between age, period, and cohort by substituting for one or more of these factors one or more characteristics of age groups and/or periods and/or cohorts. For example, a researcher might substitute the average years spent smoking before the age of 40 per members of cohorts as a measure of different cohorts' exposure to smoking when the outcome variable is lung cancer mortality (Preston and Wang 2006) or the relative size of the birth cohort (baby boom versus baby bust cohorts) when the outcome variable is suicide or homicide (O'Brien, Stockard, and Isaacson 1999; Stockard and O'Brien 2002a) or the total unemployment rate during different periods when the outcome variable is women's unemployment rates (Farkas 1977). Using these characteristics of factors breaks the linear dependency between age, period, and cohort; if one knows the period and the age, that does not determine the value of the relative cohort size variable, or if one knows the age category and the cohort category, it does not determine the period unemployment rate.

One advantage of this approach to analyzing APC data is that it provides us with a "mechanism" by which age and/or period and/or cohort factors influence the outcome variable. That is, although the categories of age, period, and cohort tell us how the age, period, and cohort categories are associated with the outcome variable, they do not tell us why. If an analysis shows a relationship between relative cohort size and age–period-specific unemployment rates or age–period-specific mean age at first marriage or age–period-specific homicide rates, we are closer to understanding the mechanisms by which the cohort effects come about. The disadvantage is that the characteristic or characteristics used to represent a factor are not likely to capture the full effect of that factor. This is a problem in any analysis but typically is more serious in an APC analysis because to the extent that the characteristics do not capture the full effect of the factor, the effects of the other factors are likely to be seriously misspecified. The linear dependency of the age, period, and cohort factors means that to the extent that the characteristics do not capture the linear effects of a factor, the other factor (or factors) takes credit for its linear effects.

6.2 Characteristics for One Factor

6.2.1 Basic Model

The most common model in the literature involves using a single characteristic for one of the factors. Typically in the literature that characteristic has been a cohort characteristic, for example, relative cohort size (Kahn and Mason 1987), cohort exposure to lead (McCall and Land 2004), or cohort smoking behavior (Preston and Wang 2006). Rarely have researchers used more than a single characteristic to represent a factor, although O'Brien, Stockard, and Isaacson (1999) and Savolainen (2000) used two cohort characteristics, and Winship and Harding (2008) used multiple characteristics for multiple factors.

Table 6.1 shows effect coding for the intercept, and age, period, and cohort factors when there are three ages, three periods, and five cohorts. Regressing any one of the column independent variables (age1, age2, ..., coh4) on the other column variables results in the $R^2 = 1.00$. This indicates linear dependency for any one of the categorical variables with the other categorical variables and the intercept. If relative cohort size (see RCS column in Table 6.1) is regressed on the age- and period-effect-coded variables, then R^2 is .48, indicating that this cohort characteristic is *not linearly dependent* on the other two factors. This is what it means in a regression that knowing the values of all but one of the independent variables does not determine the value of the remaining independent variable.

TABLE 6.1

Age–Period–Cohort Characteristic Model Using Effect Coding for a 3 × 3 Age–Period Matrix

Age	Period	Cohort	RCS	Int	age1	age2	per1	per2	coh1	coh2	coh3	coh4
20–24	2000	1975–79	10.60	1	1	0	1	0	0	0	1	0
25–29	2000	1970–74	10.82	1	0	1	1	0	0	1	0	0
30–34	2000	1965–69	11.72	1	−1	−1	1	0	1	0	0	0
20–24	2005	1980–84	10.82	1	1	0	0	1	0	0	0	1
25–29	2005	1975–79	10.6	1	0	1	0	1	0	0	1	0
30–34	2005	1970–74	10.82	1	−1	−1	0	1	0	1	0	0
20–24	2010	1985–89	10.58	1	1	0	−1	−1	−1	−1	−1	−1
25–29	2010	1980–84	10.82	1	0	1	−1	−1	0	0	0	1
30–34	2010	1975–79	10.6	1	−1	−1	−1	−1	0	0	1	0

X-Matrix spans columns Int through coh4.

Although the factor-characteristic model could be written for age characteristics, period characteristics, or cohort characteristics, Equation (6.1) is written for the APC characteristic model with two cohort characteristics:

$$Y_{ij} = \mu + \alpha_i + \pi_j + \chi_1 + \chi_2 + \epsilon_{ij}. \tag{6.1}$$

Y_{ij} is the outcome value for the ith age group and jth period, μ is the intercept, α_i represents ith age group, π_j represents the jth period (the age- and period-effect-coded categories each has a reference category), and the coefficients for the two cohort characteristics are represented by χ_1 and χ_2. The random error term is represented by ϵ_{ij} and has a mean of zero. As in Chapter 2, the discussion in this chapter includes generalized linear models.

This model can be written in matrix notation as

$$y = Xb + \epsilon, \tag{6.2}$$

where y is a vector of $I \times J$ outcome values, X is the matrix of independent variables (including the intercept), and ϵ is an $I \times J$ vector of residuals or error terms. In this model there is no problem with statistical identification, since the columns of X are not linearly dependent. In terms of the geometry of the situation, the hyperplanes intersect at a single point. There is a sense in which using characteristics for age groups and/or period and/or cohorts solves the APC identification problem and there is a sense in which it does not. It solves the identification problem in the statistical sense that no explicit constraint is necessary to identify the model. It appears to be like many other regression models: a dependent variable, some dummy variables, and one or more continuous independent variables. But, as we have seen, the APC model is somewhat special in that if we leave out one of the factors, the linear effects of that factor are "absorbed" by the other factors (see especially Chapter 5). One might say that this is a simple specification error, but in APC models this confounding of the linear effects of the left out factor is complete. In the case of factor-characteristic models, to the extent that the characteristic or characteristics do not account for the linear effects of the factor that they represent, those linear effects will be absorbed by the other two factors.[*]

It is unusual for researchers to use a characteristic for a factor other than cohorts, but Farkas (1977) used the period total unemployment rate in a study on women's age–period-specific unemployment rates. This model can be written in a manner similar to Equation (6.1), and my representation in Equation (6.4) includes two period characteristics:

$$Y_{ij} = \mu + \alpha_i + \pi_j + \pi_2 + c_k + \epsilon_{ij}. \tag{6.3}$$

The same problems exist as for Equation (6.1). If the period characteristics do not account for the linear effects of period, then the age and cohort dummy variables will absorb these effects. The result will be biased estimates of the age, period, and cohort effects. For the period–cohort–age characteristic model the same considerations apply.

6.2.2 Problem of Specifying the Linear Relationship

The linear relationships of the age effects, period effects, and cohort effects are related to each other in the following straightforward manner (Rodgers 1982:782) and are presented using my own notation:

$$t_a^* = t_a + k$$

$$t_p^* = t_p - k$$

$$t_c^* = t_c + k. \tag{6.4}$$

---

[*] My argument is different from Glenn's (2005:21–22), who recognizes the problems involved in estimating the two factors that are categorically coded when one of the factors is represented by characteristics. He emphasizes that the factor characteristics are meaningful and the factors that are categorically coded are not meaningful, and that capturing the linear effects of a factor using its factor characteristics creates problems. I basically agree with Glenn on meaningfulness, but argue that we need to capture the linear effects of the factor using the characteristics. There are two reasons for this: (1) to the extent that these linear effects are captured, better estimates of the effects of the categorically coded factors are obtained and (2) the linear component of the factor measured by the factor characteristic or characteristics is likely to be substantively important. Glenn and I both recognize the problem of multicollinearity.

Here t_a, t_p, and t_c are the linear trends of the coefficients under one constraint and t_a^*, t_p^*, and t_c^* are the linear trends under a different constraint.[*] If the original solution has t_a as the linear trend for the age effects and the second solution (t_a^*) has a slope that is k units greater than that for t_a, then the slope for the second solution for periods (t_p^*) has a trend that is k less than the trend for the original solution, and the slope for the second solution for cohorts (t_c^*) has a trend that is k units greater than trend for the original solution. Changing the constraint changes the slope of all of the coefficients for all of the factors in this systematic manner.

This relationship has major implications for the interpretation of APC analyses in general and perhaps more subtly for the factor-characteristics approach described in this chapter. It is sometimes recommended that a way around the APC identification problem is to drop one of the three factors from the analysis. This might be done on theoretical/substantive grounds or it might be done because when two factors are entered into the equation the model fits the data almost as well as when all three factors are included in the equation. The rationale is that the third factor is not needed, since it does not improve the fit of the model. Dropping one of the factors from the analysis should be done with the realization that once two factors are included in the equation, they account for the linear effects of the third factor. Then when the third factor is added to the equation, the only variance left for it to account for are the deviations of its effects around the linear trend of its coefficients.

Equation (6.4) shows why the two factors in the model absorb any linear effects of the factor left out of the model. This holds whether the age, period, and cohort effects are coded linearly or as categorical variables. Imagine that the slope (trend over time) of the coefficients for the data-generating parameters for period is 2.0, but the researcher constrains the slope of period to be zero for theoretical/substantive reasons or she decides to drop the period factor from the analysis,[†] then the trend for age will be 2.0 greater than that for the generating parameters and the trend in the cohort coefficients will be 2.0 greater than that for the generating parameters. The individual age and cohort coefficients will be biased accordingly.

When one or more characteristics are used for one of the factors the situation is somewhat different, because that does not force the trend in that

---

[*] In Chapter 4 we considered t_a, t_p, and t_c as the slopes for the original solution and the slopes for the new solution were $t_a + s(v_{2a} - sv_{1a})$, $t_p + s(v_{2p} - sv_{1p})$, and $t_c + s(v_{2c} - sv_{1c})$. The distances between the adjacent null vector elements are the same in magnitude, but the trends of the null vector elements for age and cohort are in the same direction and for period in the opposite direction as those for age and cohort. If we express the magnitude (absolute values) of the added elements for the new solutions as k, we can write equation (6.4).

[†] As pointed out in Chapter 2, we do not control the relationships of the other two factors for the deviations of the period coefficients from linearity when we do not include the period factor in the analysis. The linear effects of period are absorbed by the other two factors. If we constrain the trend of periods to be zero with a zero linear trend constraint, the deviations from linearity of the period effects are controlled and any linear effects for period are absorbed by the other two factors.

factor to be zero. If, for example, the characteristics used are for cohorts, then to the extent that the cohort characteristics capture the linear effect of the cohort parameters that generated the outcome values, the age and period estimates will reflect the age and period parameters that generated the outcome values (at least their trends will). If they were to approximately provide the correct trend for cohorts then the age and period effects would not get credit for those linear effects of cohorts. Unfortunately, the extent to which the cohort characteristics capture the linear trend in the cohort parameters that generated the outcome values cannot be assessed without resorting to outside information (substantive knowledge).*

6.3 Characteristics for Two or More Factors

Having a model with characteristics for two factors or more is almost unheard of in APC modeling. The only example that I know of is that of Winship and Harding (2008), and they use a structural equation modeling approach and set their method within the framework of Pearl's (2000) causal analysis. Winship and Harding also use multiple characteristics for many of the factors in their models. They advocate specifying the mechanisms (characteristics) through which age, period, and cohorts operate and note that "[b]y adding these variables to the model identification is often possible" (2008:363). Importantly they note: "In general, it is necessary to fully specify the mechanisms with only one of the APC variables." That argument is the same as in the previous section; if the researcher can fully specify both the linear and nonlinear effects of only one of the APC factors, then the entire model is correctly specified.

Although Winship and Harding's (2008) model is intriguing, I will not provide an empirical example of their model. Instead, I follow the logic of the factor-characteristic approach and present an empirical example of using factor-characteristics models that involve more than a single factor. This provides insights into the advantages and disadvantages of such models while situating them within the general framework of this chapter rather than within the framework of structural equation modeling.

As noted earlier, two advantages of the factor-characteristic approach are that the model is statistically identified and, as Winship and Harding (2008)

---

* Even if one were able to find characteristics that estimate the linear effect of the coefficients in the factor right in terms of the trend in the coefficients that generated the outcome values, it would not produce "fully" unbiased estimates of the generating parameters for the coefficients of the other two factors. To accomplish that, cohort characteristics that modeled both the linear and the nonlinear cohort effects correctly would be needed. Note that the factor-characteristic solution is not one of the solutions on the line of solutions that characterizes the best fitting solutions when the age, period, and cohort categorical variables are used.

point out, the "mechanisms" that make period and cohort (in this case) relevant are clearly shown and their effects measured. For someone who wants to estimate (for example) the age effects and uses a model that contains period characteristics and cohort characteristics, the problem is that the two factors operationalized using characteristics rather than categorical variables may only be partially controlled for the period and cohort effects. If that is the case, then the age effects are not well measured. Someone might argue that this is the problem with the APC analyst's futile quest (Glenn 1976): the focus on wanting to know (for example) the age-distribution controlling for period and cohort effects. On the other hand, this does not seem to be an unreasonable question. As shown in the concluding chapter, the answer to such a question may be approximated, which is all that many researchers expect out of empirical analyses.

6.4 Variance Decomposition for Factors and for Factor Characteristics

As discussed in Chapter 5, when only two of the three factors (age, period, or cohort) are in the model, they account not only for the variance associated with those two factors, but for any variance accounted for by the linear relationship between the coefficients of the third factor and the dependent variable. This section focuses on how to assess the amount of this unique variance that can be explained by the characteristics for this third factor. The simplest form of this variance partitioning is presented next (the description is brief, since some of this material was covered in Chapter 5).

The researcher runs a constrained regression model containing all of the categorical variables for the three factors. That model fits the data as well as possible using the age, period, and cohort coding. R^2 is the same for models that use any of the just identified constraints. Then the model is run with only two of the factors and the difference in R^2 provides an estimate of the unique proportion of variance in the dependent variable that is accounted for by this third factor. This addition to the proportion of the variance accounted for is referred to as the unique proportion of variance accounted for by this factor, because any variance associated with the linear trend in this factor is accounted for by the other two factors. It is the variance associated with what is often referred to as the Type II sums of squares. Then the two-factor model is run with the characteristics for the third factor added and R^2 is determined. Using, for example, cohorts characteristics to code the cohort factor, the percentage of the unique variance associated with cohorts that is accounted for by the cohort characteristics is

$$\left[\left(R^2_{apcc} - R^2_{ap}\right)\big/\left(R^2_{apc} - R^2_{ap}\right)\right] \times 100, \tag{6.5}$$

where *apc* represent a model with the age, period, and cohort categorical variables; *ap* represents a model with the age and period categorical variables, and *apcc* represents a model with the age and period categorical variables and the cohort characteristics.

6.5 Empirical Examples: Age–Period-Specific Suicide Rates and Frequencies

For an empirical example age–period-specific suicide rates (and counts) in the United States for the age groups 10–14 to 70–74 and the time span from 1930 to 2010 are used. Relative cohort size and the percentage of the birth cohort that were born to nonmarried mothers serve as cohort characteristics. These two cohort characteristics were used by Stockard and O'Brien (2002b) to examine suicide rates for a data set that does not include the periods 2005 and 2010. They note that these two characteristics should be positively related to age–period-specific suicide rates. We will not detail their entire rationale here or the extensive references to the literature. Their general theoretical framework emphasizes social integration and social regulation. Relative cohort size (RCS) is a measure of how large a birth cohort is relative to the population of several older cohorts. In a sense it is a measure of the extent to which the cohort is a Baby Boom or Baby Bust cohort. Relatively large cohorts are seen to be disadvantaged. For example, they grow up with fewer adults per child, larger class sizes, and fewer entry-level jobs per entry-level job seeker, and they delay marriage (Easterlin 1978, 1987; O'Brien 1989).

Nonmarital births (NMB) are a measure of the percentage of the cohort that is born to mothers who are not married. We would have preferred a measure of the average number of years lived with a single parent during the ages from birth to 10 or 12, but such data are not available. There are empirical data that indicate that NMB and a measure of being reared in single-parent families are highly correlated.* Stockard and O'Brien (2002a) note that family resources are likely to be less in single-parent households. There is likely

---

* Savolainen (2000) operationalized changes in family structure as "the percentage of those in the five-year birth cohort who lived in a single-parent household from ages 5 to 9" (2000:125). He obtained these data by interpolating Public Use Micro Sample census data from 1910, 1940, 1960, 1970, 1980, and 1990. He had to interpolate values from 1911 to 1939 and for other years between decennial censuses. His measure is distinct from the measure based on the percentage of births to nonmarried mothers in each cohort, yet it correlates very highly with that measure ($r = .98$). More impressive, after first differencing both measures, the correlation is .90; that is, changes in his measure of single-parent families are highly correlated with changes in the measure of NMB used in this empirical example. (Savolainen supplied his measures to Jean Stockard and me.)

to be less supervision and monitoring of children, children in single-parent families are more likely to grow up in poverty, with less adequate medical care, and in neighborhoods that are less safe. For these and other reasons, we expect that cohorts with high percentages of nonmarital births will be more likely to be cohorts that have higher rates of suicide.

Age–period-specific suicide rates and counts in the United States for the periods 1930, 1935, ..., 2010 and for the age groups 10–14, 15–19, ..., 70–74 are used for the dependent variable in the examples of factor-characteristics models that follow. Corresponding to these 5-year age groups and periods spaced 5 years apart, the earliest cohort consists of those born between 1915 and 1919, and the most recent consist of those born between 1995 and 1999. The reason for the earliest cohort not extending further back in time is that the earliest available data on NMB for the United States resident population is for those born between 1915 and 1919. Data for that cohort is only available for 1917, 1918, and 1919. This explains the form of the data depicted in Table 6.2.

Table 6.2 presents an age–period table that is missing several of the age–period-specific entries. Since data on NMB for members of cohorts who were 15–19 years old and older in 1930 are not available, age–period-specific rates for those cohorts are not included in this table. This missing data does not change the linear dependency between age, period, and cohort. If we know the period and the age group, we can tell which of the cohorts is associated with any of the observations in this table. The line of solutions for the age, period, and cohort solutions is $b_c^0 = b_{c1}^0 + sv$, where in this case the null vector element for the intercept is 6.0. The age–period-specific suicide rates per 100,000 residents appear in the body of the table: 0.41 per 100,000 for those age 10–14 in 1930 and 14.70 per 100,000 for those age 50–54 in 1990. Data for the period unemployment rates are at the bottom of the columns corresponding to the period for which they are a period characteristic. Data for the cohort characteristics, RCS, and the percentage of the birth cohort born to nonmarried mothers are listed with their corresponding cohorts at the bottom of Table 6.2. In all of the analyses, I used effect coding for ages, periods, and cohorts, and treated the observations with missing values on NMB as missing values for all models in the analyses. That assures that the same cases are used for all of our analyses and treats the data for the first 12 cohorts as missing.[*]

Table 6.3 contains the age–period-specific population (in 1000s) for the populations on which the suicide rates are based. With these exposures, it is possible to calculate the number of suicides in each age–period-specific group and then conduct a Poisson analysis. The formula for generating the count data for each cell is Number of suicides = [(Rate per 100,000) × (Population per 1000)]/100.

---

[*] Specifying that if the value of NMB is missing the case is missing, STATA's regression program (StataCorp 2013) runs the analysis omitting the cohorts 1 through 12.

TABLE 6.2

Age–Period-Specific Rates of Suicide per 100,000 along with Period and Cohort Characteristics

Age	\multicolumn{17}{c}{Period}																
	1930	1935	1940	1945	1950	1955	1960	1965	1970	1975	1980	1985	1990	1995	2000	2005	2010
10–14	0.41	0.43	0.41	0.45	0.33	0.28	0.50	0.50	0.60	0.80	0.80	1.60	1.50	1.70	1.51	1.27	1.29
15–19		4.28	3.52	2.79	2.67	2.58	3.60	4.00	5.90	7.60	8.50	10.00	11.10	10.50	8.15	7.51	7.53
20–24			8.85	6.99	6.24	5.52	7.10	8.90	12.20	16.50	16.10	15.60	15.10	16.20	12.84	12.40	13.63
25–29				8.65	8.09	7.90	9.00	11.30	13.90	16.50	16.50	15.60	15.00	15.20	13.11	12.17	14.22
30–34					10.10	8.91	10.90	13.30	14.30	16.20	15.30	14.90	15.40	15.60	12.52	13.25	13.70
35–39						10.48	13.20	15.80	15.90	16.20	15.40	14.30	15.60	15.00	13.97	13.91	5.28
40–44							15.20	17.50	17.80	18.60	15.30	14.90	14.90	15.50	15.25	16.11	6.69
45–49								18.70	19.50	19.90	15.30	15.50	15.00	14.70	15.01	16.79	9.25
50–54									20.50	20.20	16.40	15.80	14.70	14.50	14.20	16.07	9.85
55–59										20.60	16.30	17.00	16.10	12.90	12.83	14.15	9.12
60–64											15.50	16.30	15.90	13.60	11.60	13.19	5.60
65–69												16.80	16.60	14.50	11.38	11.66	3.66
70–74													19.60	17.30	13.94	13.32	3.75
Unemployment	8.9	20.1	14.6	1.9	5.2	4.4	5.5	4.5	5	8.5	7.2	7.2	5.6	5.6	4.0	5.1	9.6

Cohort	RCS	NMB
1915–1919	13.59	2.10
1920–1924	13.33	2.57
1925–1929	12.09	2.93
1930–1934	11.62	3.92
1935–1939	10.80	4.08
1940–1944	12.34	3.63

Cohort	RCS	NMB
1945–1949	14.47	3.82
1950–1954	14.96	4.06
1955–1959	15.10	4.82
1960–1964	13.80	5.99
1965–1969	11.52	8.97
1970–1974	10.40	12.11

Cohort	RCS	NMB
1975–1979	10.07	5.59
1980–1984	10.40	19.61
1985–1989	10.49	24.54
1990–1994	10.09	25.20
1995–1999	9.65	32.56

TABLE 6.3

Age–Period-Specific Population Estimates in 1000s (Used for Exposure in Poisson Models)

Age											Period						
	1930	1935	1940	1945	1950	1955	1960	1965	1970	1975	1980	1985	1990	1995	2000	2005	2010
10–14	12040	12424	11715	10777	11144	13342	16925	19049	20853	20646	18236	17101	17191	18798	20620	20858	20395
15–19		11813	12320	10832	10600	11029	13326	16922	19231	21223	21104	18552	17754	18165	20262	21039	21770
20–24			11611	9287	11446	10310	10868	13404	16579	19317	21380	21000	19131	18136	19126	21038	21779
25–29				9784	12234	11600	10823	11226	13604	17183	19697	21758	21229	19017	19306	20066	21418
30–34					11550	12315	11905	11040	11505	14131	17754	20269	21907	21892	20540	20077	20400
35–39						11546	12481	11952	11079	11585	14080	17708	19976	22331	22660	21002	20267
40–44							11639	12391	11961	11175	11726	14055	17789	20273	22524	22861	21010
45–49								11360	12138	11778	11048	11646	13819	17469	20222	22485	22596
50–54									11161	11971	11698	10943	11367	13648	17775	19998	22109
55–59										10646	11616	11341	10473	11092	13559	17354	19517
60–64											10145	10994	10618	10049	10857	13002	16758
65–69												9432	10077	9922	9518	10131	12261
70–74													8021	8826	8852	8508	9202

Despite missing nearly half of the age–period-specific observations the least squares/best fitting solutions all lie on a line of solutions in multivariate space. That is, different just identifying constraints result in models with different estimated coefficients, but all of these are best fitting solutions. This occurs because the X-matrix is rank deficient by one. The predicted values of y are the same no matter what the constraint used to identify the model, as are the other estimable functions.

The suicide rates are from U.S. Department of Health, Education, and Welfare (various years) for the periods from 1930 to 1995, and for the final three periods (2000, 2005, 2010) they were drawn from the Centers for Disease Control and Prevention (2012) online program CDC WONDER. Relative cohort size is measured as the percentage of the United States resident population age 10–59 who are 10–14 when the cohort is 10–14 years old. I would have preferred a measure focusing on the "15–19-year-old relative cohort size for those 15–64," but an observation would have had to be eliminated for the most recent cohort or a measure of relative cohort size used that differs for the final cohort.[*] These two measures of RCS, however, are quite similar in terms of their trends across time. This measure is calculated based on data drawn from census sources (United States Bureau of the Census, various years) and for the most recent periods (2000, 2005, and 2010) the Centers for Disease Control and Prevention (2012) online program CDC WONDER was used. The second cohort characteristic is the percentage of the live births in the cohort that are to nonmarried women. These data are drawn from Vital Statistics (U.S. Bureau of the Census 1946, 1990) and for the most recent cohorts (1990–1994 and 1995–1999) the data for NMB came from Martin et al. (2012). For example, the percentage of NMB for the cohort born between 1930 and 1934 was calculated by finding the mean of the percentage of NMB for 1930, 1931, 1932, 1933, and 1934.[†] The period characteristic is the percent of the civilian labor force that is unemployed. These data are for the periods 1930, 1935, …, 2010. A National Bureau of Economics Research report on the annual unemployment rate (Lebergott 1957) provided the unemployment data for the periods from 1930 to 1945 and are based on federal government data (see source data cited in that report's Table 1, p. 216). Until 1948 unemployment data reported by the federal government was for those 14 and over, and after that the measurement was for those 16 and over. The data for the periods from 1950 to 2010 came from the Bureau of Labor Statistics (2013) and are unemployment rates for those 16 years and older.[‡]

---

[*] A measure of those 15–19 for the cohort born in the 1995–1999 is not available in 2010.

[†] In one case, the 1915–1919 cohort, NMB data is not available for all of the years. For that cohort NMB data is available only for the years 1917, 1918, and 1919; these three annual percentages are averaged.

[‡] The sources cited in this paragraph have overlapping estimates of the unemployment rates for the years 1948 to 1954. The average annual unemployment rates in these sources differ by .75% with the 14 and older rates being higher on average" replace with with the 14 and older rates being higher on average by .75%.

6.6 Age–Period–Cohort Characteristics (APCC) Analysis of Suicide Data with Two Cohort Characteristics

Table 6.4 presents the results from the APCC model with two cohort characteristics.* The major aim is to show how to carefully interpret these results to convey some of the substantive meaning from these analyses. In this analysis I would suggest that the researcher should typically focus on the cohort characteristics: their size, direction, statistical significance, and contribution to accounting for the variance uniquely associated with cohorts. For the ordinary least squares (OLS) analyses reported in Table 6.4 (left-hand columns), the dependent variable is the log of the age–period-specific suicide rate per 100,000. Examining the OLS analyses, both of these cohort characteristics are statistically significant ($p < .001$). As hypothesized they are both positive and, since the independent and the dependent variables are logged, they can be interpreted as elasticities. The coefficient for NMB means that a 1% increase in the percentage of the cohort born to nonmarried mothers is associated with a .975% increase in the age–period-specific rate of suicide controlling for the other independent variables in the model. The RCS coefficient indicates that a 1% increase in the RCS is associated with a 1.355% increase in the age–period-specific suicide rate controlling for the other independent variables in the model. These two cohort characteristics account for nearly 60% of the variance that is uniquely attributable to cohorts.†

The aforementioned results are important and substantively meaningful. These two cohort characteristics account for a meaningful portion of the variance in suicide rates associated with cohorts, and this relationship is statistically significant. Importantly, this model controls, the effects of the cohort characteristics for ages and periods. The other regression coefficients in Table 6.4 are likely to be substantively less meaningful; they need to be interpreted with caution. The major reason for the "less meaningful" label is that they are not necessarily controlled for in the linear effects of cohorts.

The results for the age–period (AP) model appear in the left-hand column of the OLS results in Table 6.4. From inspection, the results for the age effects in the APCC model appear to have a more positive trend than the age effects in the AP model. The slopes of the age effects are 0.244 for the APCC model and

---

* In the analyses in this chapter the logged age–period-specific suicide rate per 100,000 is used for the dependent variable in the OLS analyses. In the Poisson regression analyses, the age–period-specific frequency of suicide is used as the dependent variable and the age–period-specific population as the exposure.

† The percentage of the variance uniquely associated with cohorts is 1.46%, which is obtained subtracting the R^2 associated with a model that contains just the age and period effects (.9693) from the R^2 for a model that contains the age, period, and cohort effects with a single constraint (.9839): $.9839 − .9693 = .0146$. The model with these two cohort characteristics and ages and periods has an R^2 of .9780, so these cohort characteristics account for .0087 (= .9780 − .9693) of R^2. The percentage of the variance uniquely associated with cohorts that the cohort characteristics account for is 59.59% [= (.0087/.0146) × 100].

TABLE 6.4

Age–Period and Age–Period–Cohort Characteristic Analyses of Age–Period-Specific Suicide (Rates and Counts)

Independent Variables	Ordinary Least Squares		Poisson Regression	
	Age–Period Model	APCC Model	Age–Period Model	APCC Model
10–14	−2.510***	−3.323***	−2.410***	−2.834***
15–19	−0.482***	−1.157***	−0.437***	−0.790***
20–24	0.162**	−0.379***	0.152***	−0.131***
25–29	0.245***	−0.149*	0.197***	−0.005
30–34	0.282***	0.031	0.214***	0.089***
35–39	0.325***	0.209***	0.260***	0.202***
40–44	0.371***	0.386***	0.329***	0.334***
45–49	0.373***	0.518***	0.363***	0.431***
50–54	0.340***	0.613***	0.352***	0.486***
55–59	0.280***	0.685***	0.301***	0.509***
60–64	0.191*	0.722***	0.208***	0.485***
65–69	0.155	0.815***	0.180***	0.531***
70–74	0.268 Ref†	1.029 Ref†	0.290 Ref†	0.691 Ref†
1930	−0.553**	0.452*	−0.701***	−0.179
1935	−0.357*	0.494**	−0.355***	0.093
1940	−0.371**	0.385*	−0.309***	0.068*
1945	−0.438***	0.177	−0.418***	−0.101***
1950	−0.480***	0.033	−0.366***	−0.113***
1955	−0.504***	−0.092	−0.361***	−0.166***
1960	−0.158*	0.125	−0.077***	0.067***
1965	0.046	0.203**	0.130***	0.212***
1970	0.235*	0.260***	0.268***	0.282***
1975	0.390***	0.287***	0.392***	0.336***
1980	0.306***	0.073	0.301***	0.177***
1985	0.382***	0.017	0.303***	0.113***
1990	0.386***	−0.114	0.303***	0.048**
1995	0.347***	−0.292**	0.265***	−0.055**
2000	0.195**	−0.589***	0.144***	−0.247***
2005	0.232***	−0.695***	0.177***	−0.293***
2010	0.342 Ref†	−0.724 Ref†	0.303 Ref†	−0.242 Ref†
Log(NMB)		0.975***		0.517***
Log(RCS)		1.355***		0.926***
Intercept	2.164***	−4.532***	−2.394***	−6.481***

* Significant at the .05 level; ** significant at the .01 level; *** significant at the .001 level.
† The coefficients marked Ref are the reference categories for age and period in each of the models.

0.111 for the AP model representing a 0.133 increase in the slope of the age effects as we move from the AP model to the APCC model. The change in the trend as we move from the AP to the APCC model for the period effects is -0.128 (= $-0.064 - 0.064$), and the change in trend as we move from the AP to the APCC model for cohorts is 0.142.* It is not a coincidence that the signs and magnitudes of these changes are similar to those indicated in Equation (6.4).

Equation (6.4) shows the relationship between the trends of age, trends of period, and trends of cohort effects for the infinite number of solutions to the just identified APC model. Equation (6.4) is exactly true for the just identified APC model; a shift in the trend of the cohort effects is matched exactly by a shift in the trend of the age effects and a shift of the same magnitude but with opposite sign for the period effects. This approximately occurs in the present situation where the cohort effects are estimated using cohort characteristics rather than using cohort categorical variables. The trend over time for the cohort effects based on the two cohort characteristics is 0.142. That is, the slope for cohorts changes from 0 when cohorts are not in the model to 0.142 when the cohort characteristics are in the model. Adding the cohort characteristics to the AP model changes the slope of the age effects by 0.133 and the slope of the period effects by -0.128.

How valid are the estimates for the age and period effects in the APCC model? I would answer that they are generally valid estimates to the extent that the cohort characteristics in the model capture the linear effects of the cohort effects for the parameters that generated the outcome data. Assessing whether the cohort characteristics model these trends is difficult. Even if the cohort characteristics accounted for all of the variance that the cohort effects can account for in an approach that first uses an AP model, the cohort characteristics can only account for the deviations from any linear trend in the cohort effects. This variance accounted for approach does not indicate whether the cohort characteristics have accounted for the linear effects of cohorts. In Chapter 7 an APCC model is presented for which there are substantive reasons to expect a particular age distribution for the dependent variable. Adding cohort characteristics to the AP model shifts the age distribution to one that fits these strong substantive expectations very well. This provides some justification for thinking that those cohort characteristics have captured at least some of the linear effects of cohorts.

The rationale for what parts of the APCC analysis are considered substantively meaningful and to what extent for the OLS analyses are the same for the Poisson regression analyses. Examining the results in Table 6.4, the

---

* To calculate the slope of the cohort effects based on the two cohort characteristics, the logged NMB and logged RCS values for each cohort were multiplied times their respective coefficient estimates and added together. This provides an estimate of the cohort effect for each cohort. Then the trend in these cohort effects from the earliest to the most recent cohort was calculated and the result was a trend of .142.

Poisson regression coefficients for both the logged values of NMB and RCS are statistically significant (p < .001). The coefficient associated with the log of NMB of .517 can be interpreted as an elasticity because this independent variable is logged and the link function used in the Poisson regression is the log link. A 1% change in NMB is associated with a .517% change in the age–period-specific expected suicide frequency. A 1% change in RCS is associated with a .926% increase in the age–period-specific expected suicide frequency controlling for the other independent variables in the model. The elasticities for the OLS and Poisson regression are not the same,[*] but are both interpretable as percentage change in the outcome variable for a 1% change in the independent variable. The likelihood ratio chi-square associated with the improvement of fit of adding these two cohort characteristics to the AP model is 636.08 with two degrees of freedom (p < .001). These two cohort characteristics certainly improve the fit of the model, and they are both controlled for age and period effects using categorically coded variables. This is a strong control for the age and period effects.

Again the relationship of the age and period coefficients to the parameters that generated the outcome data is in some doubt. There seems to be a more positive slope in the age coefficients in the APCC model than in the AP model. This is not a problem if the parameters that generated the outcome data also have age coefficients with a more positive slope than exhibited in the coefficients from the AP model. The question is whether with these two cohort characteristics in the model, the cohort slope is similar to that for the parameters that generated the outcome values. The slope for cohorts in the AP model is zero. The slope of the cohort effects over time as estimated by the two cohort characteristics in the APCC Poisson regression model is 0.072. The change in the slope for the age effects from the AP model to the APCC model is 0.069. As expected it shifts in a positive direction as does the slope for the cohorts and, as expected, the period effects shift in a negative direction –0.065. Again each of these changes in trend is of approximately the same absolute value.

6.7 Age–Cohort–Period Characteristics (ACPC) Analysis of the Suicide Data with Two Period Characteristics

The age–cohort–period characteristics (ACPC) model presented in this section is perhaps not as well motivated as the aforementioned APCC model. While I do expect that the period unemployment rate will be positively related to the age–period-specific rates of suicide, I have no expectation

---

[*] The confidence intervals for relative cohort size overlap for the OLS and Poisson analyses, but those for nonmarital birth do not overlap.

that it will account for most of the period effects. A dummy variable for the Vietnam War era period is added to this model, since it was a war that deeply divided the nation and corresponded with much social unrest. It is an exploratory variable that should probably be positively related to suicide rates. The periods 1965, 1970, and 1975 are coded as 1 on this variable and the remaining periods as 0.

Again, the strategy is to emphasize what can be concluded with some confidence from the ACPC model. The results for the OLS analyses in Table 6.5 show that a 1% increase in the period unemployment rate is associated with a .126% increase in the age–period-specific suicide rate (p < .05) controlling for the other independent variables in the model. The dummy variable for the Vietnam era has a strong positive association with the age-period-specific suicide rate. The Vietnam era is associated with a .298 increase in the logged age–period-specific suicide rate (p < .001). Importantly these relationships for the period characteristics are controlled for age and cohort effects. In terms of variance accounted for, the full APC model with one constraint accounts for 98.39% of the variance in the logged age–period-specific suicide rates. The age–cohort (AC) model accounts for 94.93% of the variance, and the ACPC model accounts for 96.24% of the variance. The two period characteristics account for 37.86% {= [(96.24 − 94.93)/(98.39 − 94.93)] × 100} of the variance that is unique to periods.

In this analysis the age and cohort coefficients are quite similar when we compare the results from the ACPC model and the AC model. This is to be expected because the period trend based on the two period characteristics is only −0.0026, meaning that the trend in the period effects has changed from 0 for the AC model to −0.0026 in the ACPC model. The trends are almost identical. Again the question is whether this trend represents the trend in the period effects that generated the outcome values. If it does, we would have some confidence in the age and cohort estimates as representing the parameters that generated the outcome values. Because of this slight trend in the estimated period effects based on the period characteristics, there is only a slight change in the age and cohort slopes from the AC model to the ACPC model: both small and positive.

Substantively, the results from the Poisson regression are similar (as they typically will be with large event counts and if the rates for the OLS analysis are logged). The two period characteristics—logged unemployment rates and Vietnam era—are both statistically significant at the .001 level. The coefficient for the logged unemployment rate can be interpreted as an elasticity: a 1% increase in the unemployment rate is associated with a .172% increase in the expected frequency of the age–period-specific suicide rate. The coefficient for Vietnam means that being in the Vietnam era is associated with a .254 change in the log of the expected age–period-specific suicide frequency. The likelihood ratio chi-square associated with the addition of these two period characteristics to the model is 2759.70 with two degrees of freedom (p < .001). As with the OLS analysis, the coefficients for the age and cohort effects are

TABLE 6.5

Age–Cohort and Age–Cohort–Period Characteristic Analyses of Age–Period-Specific Suicide (Rates and Counts)

Independent Variables	Ordinary Least Squares		Poisson Regression	
	Age–Cohort Model	ACPC Model	Age–Cohort Model	ACPC Model
10–14	−2.901***	−2.932***	−2.615***	−2.669***
15–19	−0.801***	−0.833***	−0.577***	−0.630***
20–24	−0.100	−0.123*	0.046***	0.004
25–29	0.046	0.031	0.115***	0.093***
30–34	0.157*	0.132*	0.155***	0.138***
35–39	0.283***	0.257***	0.226***	0.215***
40–44	0.428***	0.399***	0.337***	0.324***
45–49	0.497***	0.467***	0.403***	0.385***
50–54	0.522***	0.515***	0.429***	0.424***
55–59	0.503***	0.523***	0.411***	0.429***
60–64	0.434***	0.496***	0.339***	0.399***
65–69	0.416***	0.482***	0.316***	0.389***
70–74	0.516 Ref[†]	0.587 Ref[†]	0.415 Ref[†]	0.499 Ref[†]
1915–19	−0.263**	−0.315***	−0.098***	−0.164***
1920–24	−0.300***	−0.347***	−0.119***	−0.176***
1925–29	−0.344***	−0.375***	−0.148***	−0.193***
1930–34	−0.382***	−0.403***	−0.200***	−0.242***
1935–39	−0.408***	−0.445***	−0.226***	−0.271***
1940–44	−0.332***	−0.370***	−0.160***	−0.199***
1945–49	−0.215**	−0.256***	−0.102***	−0.129***
1950–54	−0.088	−0.130	0.009	0.004
1955–59	−0.011	−0.030	0.050***	0.072***
1960–64	0.053	0.062	0.069***	0.112***
1965–69	0.064	0.115	0.050***	0.100***
1970–74	0.242*	0.295**	0.107***	0.162***
1975–79	0.245*	0.303**	0.053***	0.111***
1980–84	0.331*	0.388**	0.076***	0.128***
1985–89	0.381*	0.441**	0.113***	0.145***
1990–94	0.425*	0.465**	0.141***	0.153***
1995–99	0.601 Ref[†]	0.600 Ref[†]	0.385 Ref[†]	0.385 Ref[†]
Log(unemployment)		0.126*		0.172***
Vietnam		0.298***		0.254***
Intercept	2.555***	2.302***	−2.119***	−2.454***

* Significant at .05 level; ** significant at the .01 level; *** significant at the .001 level.
† The coefficients marked Ref are the reference categories for age and cohort in each of the models.

quite similar for the AC and ACPC analyses. The trend in the period effects over time based on the two period characteristics in the Poisson regression model is –0.0035. This small shift in the trend for periods does not greatly affect the trends of the age and cohort coefficients in moving from the AC model to the ACPC model.

6.8 Age–Period–Characteristics–Cohort Characteristics Model

As noted in the introduction to this chapter, it is unusual for a researcher to have characteristics for more than one of the factors in a factor-characteristic model. One reason is the difficulty in finding convincing characteristics that plausibly capture the effects of even a single factor let alone two such factors. A second reason is noted by Winship and Harding (2008:363) who state: "In general, it is necessary to fully specify the mechanisms with only one of the APC variables." If we could specify one of the factors fully, including its linear effects, then we could obtain unbiased estimates of the age, period, and cohort effects. It is not at all clear that specifying mechanisms for two of the factors would provide better estimates of the age, period, and cohort effects. It would, however, help establish some of the mechanisms that might account for the effects of these factors.

In this section a model is presented in which age is represented by the effect-coded categorical variables, and the two characteristics for periods and the two for cohorts are those from the two earlier analyses. As Table 6.6 shows, all four of the characteristics are statistically significant at the .01 level or less. For the OLS analysis, the log of NMB has an elasticity of .460, meaning that a 1% change in this variable is related to a .460% increase in the age–period-specific suicide rate ($p < .001$), controlling for the other independent variables in the model. The coefficient associated with RCS indicates that a 1% change in relative cohort size is associated with a .757% increase in the age–period-specific suicide rate ($p < .001$). The first of the period characteristics indicates that a 1% increase in unemployment is associated with a .153% increase in the age–period-specific suicide rate ($p < .01$), controlling for the other independent variables in the model. Being in the Vietnam era (rather than in other periods) is associated with a .271 increase in the logged age–period-specific suicide rate ($p < .001$), controlling for the other independent variables in the model.

Interpreting the coefficients associated with characteristics in models with characteristics for two factors is different than interpreting the coefficients associated with characteristics in models with characteristics for only a single factor. In the model with characteristics for only one factor the

TABLE 6.6

Age and Age–Period–Characteristic, Cohort Characteristic Analyses of
Age–Period-Specific Suicide (Rates and Counts)

Independent Variables	Ordinary Least Squares		Poisson Regression	
	Age Only	APCCC Model	Age Only	APCCC Model
10–14	−2.709***	−2.917***	−2.515***	−2.652***
15–19	−0.647***	−0.821***	−0.507***	−0.631***
20–24	0.023	−0.109	0.106***	0.007
25–29	0.136	0.049	0.163***	0.102***
30–34	0.215*	0.147*	0.193***	0.156***
35–39	0.309**	0.267***	0.257***	0.235***
40–44	0.417***	0.394***	0.350***	0.332***
45–49	0.460***	0.457***	0.403***	0.389***
50–54	0.453***	0.495***	0.404***	0.415***
55–59	0.402**	0.500***	0.357***	0.411***
60–64	0.304*	0.472***	0.254***	0.3671***
65–69	0.269*	0.473***	0.219***	0.376***
70–74	0.368 Ref[†]	0.593 Ref[†]	0.316 Ref[†]	0.492 Ref[†]
Log(NMB)		0.460***		0.260***
Log(RCS)		0.757		0.670***
Log(unemployment)		0.153**		0.171***
Vietnam		0.271***		0.230***
Intercept	2.363***	−1.592**	−2.180***	−5.224***

* Significant at .05 level; ** significant at the .01 level; *** significant at the .001 level.
[†] The coefficients marked Ref are the reference category for age in each of the models.

characteristics are controlled for the other factors using categorical variables. For example, for the period-characteristic model the characteristics are controlled for the effects of age and cohort categorical variables. In the current model with characteristics for cohorts and periods, the period characteristics are controlled for age effects using categorical variables but not for cohort effects using categorical variables. The cohort characteristics are controlled for age effects using categorical variables but not for period effects using categorical variables. It makes these characteristic coefficients less meaningful unless both sets of characteristics are very good estimates of the effects of the factors.

In terms of variance accounted for the procedure is similar to that for the situation in which there are characteristics for only a single factor. As before, the proportion of the variance accounted for by the full model with all three factors and one constraint is .9839. When only the age categorical variables are in the model the proportion of the variance accounted for is .9044 and when we add the period and cohort characteristics to this model the proportion of the variance accounted for is .9557. The proportion of variance in the model that is unique to period and cohort is .0795 (= 9839 − .9044) and the amount of that variance accounted for by the period and cohort characteristics is .0513 (= .9557 − .9044). The percentage of the variance that is uniquely associated with periods and cohorts that is accounted for by these characteristics is 64.53% [= (.0513/.0795) × 100].

The results from the Poisson regression models for the cohort and period characteristics are similar. The logged independent variables can be interpreted as elasticities: a 1% increase in NMB is associated with a .260% increase in the age–period-specific expected frequency of suicides; a 1% increase in RCS is associated with a .670% increase in the age–period-specific expected frequency of suicides; a 1% increase in the unemployment rate is associated with a .171% increase in the age–period-specific frequency of suicides controlling for all of the other independent variables in the model. The coefficient for Vietnam era indicates that being in the Vietnam era rather than not being in that era is associated with an increase of .230 in the logged age–period-specific expected frequency of suicide. All of these are statistically significant relationships (p < .001).

I do not assume that the age coefficients are reliable estimates of the age parameters that generated the values of the age–period-specific suicide rates for either the OLS or Poisson regression models. For them to be accurate estimates, the linear effects of cohorts would need to be captured by the two cohort characteristics and the linear effects of periods would need to be captured by the two period characteristics. Further, there is no assurance that the characteristic coefficients themselves have been controlled for the other factor represented by factor characteristics.

6.9 Approaches Based on Factor Characteristics and Mechanism

As noted earlier, the mechanism-based approach of Winship and Harding (2008), which is specifically designed to include multiple characteristics for multiple factors, is not used with empirical data in this chapter. That approach uses structural equation modeling and is presented within the causal modeling framework of Pearl (2000). That approach would have led us too far afield from the main approach of this chapter and those featured in this book. But the use of multiple characteristics for multiple factors in the last section highlights some of the interpretational problems that are likely to be encountered using the mechanism-based approach.

One problem for both the factor-characteristic approach and the mechanism-based approach is finding a set of characteristics that fully captures the effects of each of the factors modeled by characteristics. Imagine that a single factor is modeled by characteristics and that factor is cohorts. The effects of the cohort characteristics are controlled fully for age and period effect categorical variables—in such a way that the form of the relationship between age and period and the dependent variable is very flexible (given the categorical coding). We will not have much confidence in the age and period categorical effects estimates unless we think that the cohort characteristics capture at least the linear effects of cohorts. If the cohort characteristics capture the linear effects of the cohort parameters that generated the outcome data, then our estimates of the age and period categorical effects should be quite good.

The cohort characteristics in this situation are meaningfully interpreted as the relationship between these characteristics of cohorts and the outcome variable controlling for the other two factors and any other cohort characteristics in the model; and here, the controls for age and period effects are quite strong. These characteristics generally should not be interpreted as an unbiased estimate of the cohort effects that generated the outcome values. When there are factor characteristics for more than a single factor, the coefficients associated with the characteristics do not have these strong controls for the other two factors.

In general using fit to gauge a factor-characteristic model is problematic. The models often fit extremely well. It is not unusual for two of the categorically coded variables to account for more than 90% of the variance in the dependent variable. For the suicide data in this chapter the categorically coded age factor by itself accounted for over 90% of the variance in the logged age–period-specific suicide rates. An APCC model in which the cohort characteristics accounted for all of the unique variance possible (the deviations of the cohort effects from the linear trend in the cohort effects) could still be seriously misspecified in that its linear trend did not match the linear trend in the parameters that generated the outcome values.[*] This is like the infinite number of solutions on the line of solutions that fit the model equally well but can have quite different parameter estimates.

Winship and Harding's (2008) mechanism-based approach has not been employed much in the published literature. It is that use and engagement that will help researchers fully evaluate the mechanism-based approach. The approach is innovative enough that the nuances of its advantages and disadvantages are difficult to gauge at this point. It will need, however, to address the issues raised in this and the previous section; perhaps especially, the less stringent controls for age effects, period effects, and cohort effects when multiple factors are represented by characteristics.

---

[*] To account for all of the unique variance associated with cohorts, what is necessary is to account for the deviations from the linear trend and not necessarily the linear trend component itself.

6.10 Additional Features and Analyses of Factor-Characteristic Models

There are many other features that can be applied to a factor-characteristic model. O'Brien (2000) notes there are three types of control variables in APCC models. The factor characteristics themselves control the other independent variables in the model for the factor-characteristic effects. The categorical variables for age and period are fixed effects and control for any factors that are associated with age that do not change over periods and any factors that are associated with periods that do not change over ages. Variables that vary over age and period and cohort can be controlled for. O'Brien labels these as "contemporaneous controls." They are age–period-specific variables such as the age–period–specific unemployment rate or the sex ratio that vary by age and period. Note that this is different from treating the unemployment rate as a period characteristic where it is the same for all cells within a period. These "contemporaneous controls" can take on different values for each cell of the table. The age–period-specific unemployment rate or sex ratio can be entered into the analysis as a control variable (and, of course, their substantive effects examined). These variables (that take up only a single degree of freedom) have seldom been used in APC analysis. Interactions between different cohort characteristics and periods or age groups can also be added to an APCC model allowing for nonadditive effects (O'Brien 2000).

Different methods of analysis can be used not just standard OLS and generalized linear models. Seemingly unrelated regression (SUR) models appear to be underused. O'Brien and Stockard (2006) used a SUR model for age–period-specific rates of suicide and homicide in the United States. The model involves an APCC model for homicides victimization and for suicides. It allows residuals for the two models to be correlated and estimates these correlations. The model is also statistically more efficient than running separate models for homicide and suicide. In their application O'Brien and Stockard (2006) show that the two cohort characteristics (NMB and RCS) decreased the correlation between the residuals substantially when they were entered into an equation that contained only the age and period categorical variables, but that there were still other factors not in the model that were needed to account for this correlation between the residuals. In areas where APC data are available by gender, race, and other characteristics, SUR models are potentially quite useful.

6.11 Conclusions

Factor-characteristic models avoid the statistical identification problem faced by APC modelers but at a cost. This approach provides a solution that does not fall on the line of solutions discussed in Chapter 2, and these solutions have been the focus of interest for most APC modelers whether by design or not. It is probably for this reason (as noted at the head of this chapter) that Glenn (2005:21) states in the context of factor-characteristic models: "It is extremely important to keep in mind, however, that these models are not true APC models (although they are sometimes represented as such) and in no sense provide a solution to the age-period-cohort conundrum." Glenn goes on to note that: "It is unlikely that cohort effects on any dependent variable result only from the cohort-characteristics included in the models, and any remaining cohort-effects are confounded in the model estimates with age and period effects." I have explicated and emphasized this final point in this chapter, and have shown why this is the case.

I argue for factor characteristics that capture the linear trends in the categorical coefficients for the factor that approximates the trend in the parameters that generated the outcome data. Otherwise the linear trend that should be associated with that factor is absorbed by the other factors making their estimates inaccurate. This is contrary to the advice of Glenn (2005:22) who states: "[I]t is also important to avoid independent variables that bear a strong linear relationship with the omitted APC variable." It is true that these variables will be highly correlated, but this "strong linear relationship" is necessary to control the effects of the categorically coded factors for the linear effects of the characteristic-coded factor.

This understanding of the relationship between factors in the factor-characteristic approach is crucial for the interpretation of the results. The factor characteristics in the model with one factor having characteristics and two factors represented by their categorically coded variables are interpretable as the characteristics' effects controlling for the other two factor effects. This interpretation seems straightforward and "meaningful." This is not the case for the two factors that are measured by sets of categorical variables. To the extent that the factor characteristics do not capture the effects of the factor coded with characteristics, then the categorical effects of the other two factors are confounded with the linear effects of the third factor and to that extent are not "meaningful."

As we add characteristics for additional factors, the controls provided by these factors for the age effects and/or period effects and/or cohort effects become less strong, since the controls provided by the categorical representation of the factor effects are only approximated by the factor characteristics. For example, in the age–period–characteristic–cohort characteristic model the age effects may not be adequately controlled for the period effects and the cohort effects. Unless the researcher has very excellent factor characteristics for multiple factors, it may be preferable to model just the single factor with the best characteristics.[*] In our first empirical example we know, at least,

---

[*] Others might argue that knowing about the mechanisms is so important that having characteristics for multiple factors is more important than the enhanced controls offered by the categorical coding of factors.

that the relationship between the cohort characteristics (relative cohort size and the percentage of nonmarital births) and suicide rates is controlled for age effects and period effects, and we can concentrate on interpreting the relationship of those cohort characteristics to the age–period-specific rates of suicide.

References

Bureau of Labor Statistics. 2013. Labor force participation statistics from the Current Population Survey (Series LNS 14000000). Online database (generated on May 4, 2013).

Centers for Disease Control and Prevention. 2012. Underlying cause of death 1999-2010 on CDC WONDER. Online Database, released 2012, http://wonder.cdc.gov/ucd-icd10.html (accessed at July 2, 2013).

Easterlin, R. 1978. What will 1984 be like? Socioeconomic implications of recent twists in age structure. *Demography* 15:397–421.

Easterlin, R. 1987. *Birth and Fortune: The Impact of Numbers on Personal Welfare*. Chicago: University of Chicago Press.

Farkas, G. 1977. Cohort, age, and period effects upon the employment of white females: Evidence for 1957–1968. *Demography* 14:33–42.

Glenn, N.D. 1976. Cohort analysts' futile quest: Statistical attempts to separate age, period, and cohort effects. *American Sociological Review* 41:900–904.

Glenn, N.D. 2005. *Cohort Analysis* (2nd edition). Thousand Oaks, California: Sage.

Kahn, J.R., and W.M. Mason. 1987. Political alienation, cohort size, and the Easterlin hypothesis. *American Sociological Review* 52:155–69.

Lebergott, S. 1957. Annual estimates of unemployment in the United States. National Bureau of Economic Research.

Martin, J.A., B.E. Hamilton, S.J. Ventura, et al. 2012. Births: Final data for 2010. *National Vital Statistics Reports*, vol. 61 no. 1. Hyattsville, MD: National Center for Health Statistics.

McCall, P.L., and K.C. Land. 2004. Trends in environmental lead exposure and troubled youth, 1960–1995: An age-period-cohort-characteristic analysis. *Social Science Research* 33:339–59.

O'Brien, R.M. 1989. Relative cohort size and age-specific crime rates. *Criminology* 27:57–78.

O'Brien, R.M. 2000. Age, period, cohort characteristic models. *Social Science Research* 29:123–39.

O'Brien, R.M., and J. Stockard. 2006. A common explanation for the changing age distribution of suicide and homicide in the United States: 1930 to 2000. *Social Forces* 84:1539–57.

O'Brien, R.M., J. Stockard, and L. Isaacson. 1999. The enduring effects of cohort size and percent of nonmarital births on age-specific homicide rates, 1960–1995. *American Journal of Sociology* 104:1061–95.

Pearl, J. 2000. *Causality: Models, Reasoning, and Inference*. Cambridge, UK: Cambridge University Press.

Preston, S.H., and H. Wang. 2006. Sex mortality differences in the United States: The role of cohort smoking patterns. *Demography* 43:631–46.

Rodgers, W.L. 1982. Estimable functions of age, period, and cohort effects. *American Sociological Review* 47:774–87.

Savolainen, J. 2000. Relative cohort size and age-specific arrest rates: A conditional interpretation of the Easterlin effect. *Criminology* 38:117–36.

StataCorp. 2013. *Stata Statistical Software: Release 13*. College Station, TX: StataCorp LP.

Stockard, J., and R.M. O'Brien. 2002a. Cohort effects on suicide rates: International variations. *American Sociological Review* 67:854–72.

Stockard, J., and R.M. O'Brien. 2002b. Cohort variations and changes in age-specific suicide rates over time: Explaining variations in youth suicide. *Social Forces* 81:605–42.

U.S. Bureau of the Census. Various years. Numbers 98, 114, 170, 519, 870, 1000, 1022, 1058, 1127, and for 1995–2010 data http://www.census.gov/population/estimate-extract/nation/intfile2-l.txt. *Current Population Surveys: Series P-25*. Washington D.C.: Government Printing Office.

U.S. Bureau of the Census. 1946, 1990. *Vital Statistics of the United States: Natality*. Washington D.C.: Government Printing Office.

U.S. Department of Health, Education, and Welfare, National Center for Health Statistics. Various years. *Annual Vital Health Statistics Report*, vol. 2. Washington D.C.: Government Printing Office.

Winship, C., and D.J. Harding. 2008. A mechanism based approach to the identification of age-period-cohort models. *Sociological Methods & Research* 36:362–401.

7

Conclusions: An Empirical Example

I hope that authors who cite this edition will recognize that, except under conditions that hardly ever exist, a definitive separation of age, period, and cohort effects is not just difficult, but impossible. However, I also hope that they will realize that a definitive separation of the effects is not necessary in order for cohort analysis to be useful.

N.D. Glenn (2005:vii)

7.1 Introduction

For me, delving deeply into the traditional age–period–cohort (APC) problem represents a long-time passion. As noted in the Preface, it began with a talk given by Bill Mason at the University of Oregon in 1987 or 1988. But there were also years of inactivity in this area until I began working on these models again with my colleague Jean Stockard. I had given her some data on the epidemic of youth homicide, and she thought she knew a cohort factor that might account for this phenomenon. I said I knew another one and that I knew how to test it. We were off on the most wonderful collaborative research of my career. As always my substantive interest in problems ignited my methodological interest. For me they go hand in hand. Then the work of Yang, Fu, and Land (2004) and Yang, Schulhofer-Wohl, Fu, and Land (2008) inspired an interest in the technical details of APC constrained models—the major traditional technique in the APC literature—but one that I had never used in substantive research. All this has culminated in this book.

If I am successful, diligent readers should have a reasonably deep understanding of the classic APC identification problem from both algebraic and geometric perspectives. They should see how this problem rears its unpleasant head when researchers statistically identify a model by modeling only two of the three factors, replace one or more of the factors with characteristics, or use any particular mechanical constraint. The book covers in some detail just four techniques: constrained estimation, estimable functions, variance decomposition, and factor characteristics. Together these techniques are the ones used in much of the literature that analyzes APC aggregate-level data, but they are certainly not the only ones or the majority of the different techniques that have been developed. They are, however, a reasonably unified set of techniques and provide an excellent set of tools for understanding other APC methods found in the literature and which appear from time to time in rediscovered forms or as somewhat innovative new approaches.

This concluding chapter takes a different form than such chapters in most books. I decided to present a single substantive example from an area of research in which I possess substantive expertise. This empirical example provides a plausible estimate of the relationship of age, period, and cohorts to the age–period-specific rates of homicide arrests over a 45-year period in the United States. That effort employs a combination of the techniques discussed in this book and a "sensitivity analysis" based on the line of solutions. It is in the spirit of the quote from Glenn (2005: viii) at the head of this chapter: "that a definitive separation of the effects is not necessary in order for cohort analysis to be useful."

There are some things that can be concluded with much certainty about APC models and some of their parameters. These have to do with estimable functions and include the unique variance accounted for, total variance accounted for, the predicted values of the outcome variable, deviation of effects from their linear trends, and shifts in trends within factors. There are other questions to which there are no definitive answers. To attempt to answer these questions one must rely on theory and past research for decisions about the appropriate constraint or factor characteristics to utilize. In this chapter, I show how one can use the definitive answers and use substantive knowledge combined with constrained regression and factor characteristics to provide a plausible picture of the age, period, and cohort effects.

7.2 Empirical Example: Homicide Offending

The empirical data involves homicide offenders in the United States broken down by 5-year age groups 15–19, 20–24, ..., 60–64. Data were obtained for the periods 1965, 1970, ..., 2010 and the corresponding birth cohorts are 1900–04, 1905–09, ..., 1990–94. Observations on the first three cohorts were dropped because data on two crucial cohort characteristics are lacking for these three cohorts. Data on homicide offending (number of offenders by age groups and the total U.S. population covered by reporting law enforcement agencies in each period) were drawn from *Crime in the United States* (Federal Bureau of Investigation, various years). The age–period-specific rates appear in Table 7.1.*

---

* The arrest figures from the FBI are based on the number of reporting agencies, which varies from period to period. To correct for this effect the total population of the United States for the period was divided by the number of residents in the areas reporting to the FBI in that period. This ratio was multiplied times the number of homicide arrests in each of the age groups in that period. This corrected number of age–period-specific homicides arrests was divided by the number of U.S. residents in the age–period-specific category (U.S. Bureau of the Census, various years) and multiplied by 100,000 to obtain the age–period-specific rates per 100,000 in Table 7.1.

TABLE 7.1

Age–Period-Specific Homicide Rates (per 100,000) and Values of Relative Cohort Size and Nonmarital Births for Birth Cohorts

					Period					
Age	1965	1970	1975	1980	1985	1990	1995	2000	2005	2010
15–19	9.07	17.22	17.54	18.00	16.32	35.17	35.08	14.63	13.87	10.89
20–24	15.18	23.75	25.62	23.97	21.10	29.10	31.93	18.46	18.70	13.08
25–29	14.69	20.09	21.05	18.88	16.79	18.00	16.76	10.90	11.85	8.63
30–34	11.70	16.00	15.81	15.23	12.58	12.44	10.05	6.63	6.80	5.94
35–39	9.76	13.13	12.83	12.32	9.60	9.38	7.25	5.41	4.69	4.10
40–44	7.41	10.10	10.52	8.80	7.50	6.81	5.47	3.74	3.69	2.88
45–49	5.56	7.50	7.32	6.76	5.31	5.17	3.67	2.30	3.09	2.39
50–54	4.60	5.68	4.91	4.36	4.32	3.38	2.68	1.70	1.74	1.71
55–59	3.13	4.38	3.34	3.28	3.31	2.36	2.50	0.89	1.22	1.19
60–64	2.38	2.78	2.99	2.16	1.90	1.77	1.39	0.64	0.76	0.73

Cohort Characteristics

	1915–19	1920–24	1925–29	1930–34	1935–39	1940–44	1945–49	1950–54	1955–59	1960–64
RCS	13.89	13.69	12.39	10.80	10.87	12.43	14.62	15.27	15.33	14.03
NMB	2.10	2.57	2.93	3.92	4.08	3.63	3.82	4.06	4.82	5.99

	1965–69	1970–74	1975–79	1980–84	1985–89	1990–94
RCS	11.72	10.82	10.60	10.82	10.58	10.49
NMB	8.97	12.11	15.59	19.60	24.54	30.24

The cohorts are on the main diagonals of the table. For example, the youngest age group (15–19) in the earliest period (1965) corresponds to the 10th earliest cohort and was born 1945–49. It has a homicide offense rate of 9.07 per 100,000. Five years later this cohort is in the 20–24-year-old age range and it has an age–period-specific homicide offense rate of 23.75. Relative cohort size (RCS) is the percentage of the population 15–64 who were 15–19 when the birth cohort was 15–19. It is a measure of the degree to which a cohort is a baby boom or baby bust cohort. Easterlin (1978, 1987) provides a strong rationale and empirical evidence that baby boom cohorts are disadvantaged in a number of ways: they have fewer adults per child, more crowded classrooms, fewer entry-level jobs per entry-level job seeker, delayed marriage, and delayed childbearing (Macunovich 1999; O'Brien, Stockard, and Isaacson 1999). Nonmarital births (NMB) are measured as the percentage of live births that were to nonmarried mothers for each of the cohorts. For example, for the 1980–84 cohort NMB is the mean of the percentage of births to nonmarried mothers for the years 1980, 1981, …, 1984. For the 1915–19 cohort the only data available were for the years 1917 to 1919 and its percentage is based on the average of these three years. There were no data for nonmarital births for earlier cohorts. The values of the cohort characteristics for both RCS and NMB appear at the bottom of Table 7.1. The earliest cohort for which both RCS and NMB measures are available is the cohort born between 1915 and 1919: the RCS was 13.89 and the percentage of NMB was 2.10. For the most recent cohort, the one born between 1990 and 1994, RCS was 10.49 and NMB was 30.24.

Data for calculating the RCS come from the U.S. Bureau of the Census (various years) and the Centers for Disease Control and Prevention (2012). Data on nonmarital births were drawn from the vital statistics program of the U.S. Bureau of the Census (1946, 1990) and Martin et al. (2012). For the 5-year periods from 1915 to 1990 there is a strong correlation between the percentage of NMB and the percentage of those in the 5-year birth cohorts who lived in a single-parent household from ages 5 to 9. The correlation is .98 and the correlation of first differences is .90. The data on the percentage of those living in single-parent households from age 5 to 9 was supplied by Jukka Savolainen (2000).

Stockard and O'Brien (2002) note that family resources are likely to be fewer in single-parent households. There is likely to be less supervision and monitoring of children, and children in single-parent families are more likely to grow up in poverty, with less adequate medical care, and in neighborhoods that are less safe. For these and other reasons, cohorts with high percentages of NMB will be more likely to be cohorts with higher rates of homicide offending.

The specification of the full APC model is

$$Y_{ij} = \mu + \alpha_i + \pi_j + \chi_{I-i+j} + \epsilon_{ij}. \tag{7.1}$$

Y_{ij} is the dependent variable value for the ijth cell of the age–period table; μ is the value of the intercept; α_i is the age effect of the ith age group; π_j is the period effect for the jth period; χ_{I-i+j} is the cohort effect for the $(I-i+j)$th cohort (where I is the number of age groups), and ϵ_{ij} is the error term or residual associated with the ijth cell of the age–period table. Since age, period, and cohort are categorically coded, one of the age groups, one of the periods, and one of the cohorts serve as reference groups.

7.2.1 Unique Variance and Deviations from Linearity

The first set of analyses for the homicide data involves what can be known about age, period, and cohort effects assuming that the APC full model specification in Equation (7.1) is the correct specification. They do not depend

TABLE 7.2

Unique Contribution of Cohorts, Periods, and Ages to the Variance
Accounted for in Age–Period-Specific Homicide Rates

	Degrees of Freedom	P <	F	$R^2_{increment}$
Cohorts	F(14,61)	0.0001	5.96	0.0232
Periods	F(8,61)	0.0001	26.49	0.0590
Ages	F(8,61)	0.0001	15.32	0.0341

upon the constraint chosen. A good starting point is to ascertain whether
each of the factors account for significant amounts of unique variance in the
logged homicide rates.* Table 7.2 indicates that each of the factors accounts
for a significant amount of additional variance in the dependent variable
over a model that contains only the other two factors. Remember that this
is a very stringent test, since the only *unique variance* accounted for is that due
to deviations from the linear trend of the factor. In this case, the deviations of
the cohort factors around the linear trend in these coefficients account for
an additional 2.32% of the variance in homicide rates. This is statistically
significant at the .0001 level.† Periods account for 5.90% additional variance,
and this increment in the variance is significant at the .0001 level. Age groups
account for an additional 3.41% of the variance in homicide rates, and this
increment is statistically significant at the .0001 level.

The deviations for the age coefficients from their linear trend, the deviations of period coefficients from their linear trend, and the deviations for
the cohort effects from their linear trend are estimable, and those deviations
are shown in the three graphs in Figure 7.1. The curve for the age effects
is an inverted U-shape. These deviations represent the detrended age effects.
I suspect that the linear trend of the age parameters that generated the outcome data has a negative trend, a trend that should make the age effects
display a monotonic decrease after the age group 20–24. I will provide evidence and theoretical/substantive reasons for this conjecture shortly. The
period curve is also an inverted U-shape with some small difference in this
pattern for the most recent periods. The variation of the period coefficients
around their linear trend is greater than that for the cohort coefficients; that
is, the relationship of periods to homicide offending has a stronger curvilinear component than that for cohorts. This is evident not only in Figure 7.1 but
also in Table 7.2. The cohort deviations show a U-shaped relationship over
time. But again this simply means that if there is a positive linear trend, then

---

* Note that we run all of the analyses with the earliest three cohorts missing from the analysis,
  since they are missing the data on the NMB cohort characteristic. This ensures that all of the
  analyses in this chapter use the same cases.
† The significance test is an F-test for the increment in R^2.

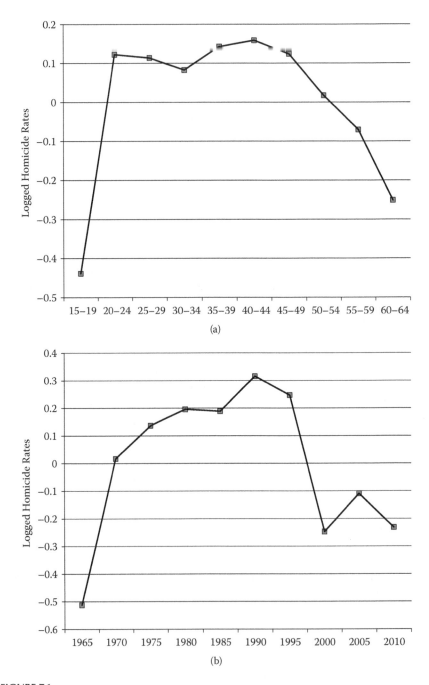

FIGURE 7.1
Deviations of the age, period, and cohort coefficients from their linear trends. (a) Age deviations from the age trend. (b) Period deviations from the period trend. (c) Cohort deviations from the cohort trend. *(continued)*

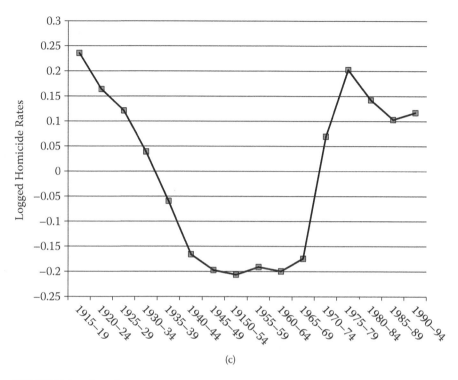

(c)

FIGURE 7.1 (continued).
Deviations of the age, period, and cohort coefficients from their linear trends. (a) Age deviations from the age trend. (b) Period deviations from the period trend. (c) Cohort deviations from the cohort trend.

the slope is relatively less positive for the early cohorts and relatively more positive for the later cohorts with the possible exception of the three most recent cohorts. If there is a negative linear trend, then the slope is relatively more negative for the earlier cohorts and relatively less negative for the more recent cohorts with the possible exception of the three most recent cohorts.

7.2.2 Constrained Regression Using the *s*-Constraint Approach

When using constrained estimation, I focus on substantive knowledge and theory to determine the constraint employed; this step is crucial for producing a constraint that is approximately "right." To facilitate setting the constraint, I introduce a procedure that allows researchers to constrain the age curve directly in the way that theory and research suggests. It also allows a flexible sensitivity analysis of the results. The constraint is set not by constraining two categorical variables to have an equal effect but by manipulating the value of s in what I will label the formula for the extended line of solutions: $b_c^0 = b_{c1}^0 + sv^*$. Here, I use the extended null vector (v^*) and the full solution for b_{c1}^0 that includes the values for the reference categories. In this case the intercept element for the null vector is 1.5.

The s-constraint approach allows the researcher to obtain any of the best fitting solutions desired. Since we know the extended null vector (v^*), we can find any of the best fitting solutions (b_c^0) using any one of the just identified constrained solutions (b_{c1}^0). I simply set up an Excel spreadsheet with one of the just identified constrained solutions as a column (b_{c1}^0) using the full solution including the coefficients for the reference categories, another column for the extended null vector (v^*), and a third column for the result (b_c^0). I then manipulated the value of s to generate different constrained solutions (b_c^0). This method works in a systematic manner allowing the researcher (in my example) to produce an age curve that is consistent with theory and substantive knowledge. It generates sets of coefficients that produce the best fitting solutions (the just identified solutions).

The first task was to produce a solution in which the age distribution matched what fairly strong substantive knowledge indicates it should be. I choose age, because it has been a central variable in criminology and there is much research available on its relationship to homicide. If a researcher could produce the correct age effects for the parameters that generated the outcome values, all of the other parameters would be correct. I set this "best substantive" solution so that it was between two extreme or boundary solutions that substantive knowledge and theory indicate are at the limits of what we would expect the age effects of homicide offending to look like.

The first boundary solution is consistent with what almost all criminologists would agree is a monotonic decrease in homicide in the age effect after the age group 20–24. This is consistent with Hirschi and Gottfredson's (1983) summary of the literature and the more biologically oriented work of Daly and Wilson (1988), Wilson and Daly (1993), and Hiraiwa-Hasegawa (2005). The second boundary solution is a bit more difficult to set. Hirschi and Gottfredson note that personal crimes peak at a later age than property crimes and this is especially true for the serious personal crimes. This means that a personal crime as serious as homicide is likely to peak in the early 20s. They also note that the age curve of offending drops off more steeply from the peak for the younger ages than for the older ages. Eisner (2003), in a review of six different European locations and from different periods of time (over a 400-year time span), finds that the age curve of violent crimes follows this pattern (see especially his Figure 10).* These findings are consistent with setting the second boundary condition such that the rates for those 15–19 years old do not exceed the rate for those 25–29 years old.

The strategy I follow is based on the goal of making a "best" estimate of the age curve based on substantive knowledge. Then I use two boundary

---

* Of course, the age effects can vary by culture.

estimates as a form of sensitivity analysis to see how this changes the period and cohort curves. I proceeded as follows. (1) Solve the APC model with a constraint (for example, age1 = age2). (2) Use the Excel spreadsheet described earlier and manipulate *s* until obtaining an age curve for the age effects that seems to best fit the substantive knowledge in the field. (3) Place boundary conditions on that estimate by manipulating *s* so that there is a monotonic drop in the homicide rates after age 20–24. I did this by systematically changing the values of *s* until such a drop "just occurred." The second boundary is one in which the age group 15–19 has a homicide offense rate that is as great as the age group 25–29 but no greater. This was found by manipulating *s* but is, of course, the same as setting age1 = age3 as a constraint. The advantage of the *s*-constraint approach is that any curve for age effects, period effects, or cohort effects can be found by choosing among the infinite number of constraints on the extended line of solutions. The boundary solutions and the "best" solution are each constrained solutions, but more importantly they are constrained solutions based on substantive knowledge and theory.

Having an age curve that is a just barely decreasing monotonically after age 25–29 and an age curve for which the 15–19- and 20–24-year-old age groups have equal age effects on the age–period-specific homicide offense rates serves as the limits in my sensitivity analysis. A major aim of this analysis is to gain some insight into the period and cohort effects. If we can obtain an accurate age curve, that should result in accurate period and cohort curves, because if the slope of the age curve was approximately correct, then the period and cohort curves should be approximately correct.

Table 7.3 presents the three sets of estimates. The first solution is the best substantive estimate (based on my reading of past research and theory); the age curve that is most consistent with substantive knowledge in the field. The next two solutions are based on substantive theory also, but represent age curves that are at the "extremes" of what substantive knowledge suggests the age curves should be. Again they are based on using a constrained solution, and *s* times the extended null vector to generate different age-effect distributions until one is found that fits the substantive boundary pattern for the age effects. This is not as haphazard as it sounds, since increasing or decreasing *s* "rotates" the solutions in a consistent direction. The first of the boundary solutions is labeled as the age4 = age5 solution. The reason for this label is that was when the monotonic decrease criterion was first met. The solution needed to be rotated until there was a decrease from the age4 to age5 to meet the monotonic decrease criterion. The constraint imposed at that value of *s* is nearly equivalent to the constraint age4 = age5. Note that for the column labeled age4 = age5, the coefficient for age 30–34 is just slightly larger than that for age 35–39. The second of the boundary solutions is labeled the age1 = age3 solution. This represents the other limit suggested by substantive research and theory that the age 25–29 category has a

TABLE 7.3

Simulated Solutions Based on Substantive Knowledge
of the Age-Effects for Homicide Offending

Effects	"Best Substantive Solution"	age 4 = age5	age1 = age3
15–19	0.466	−0.168	0.804
20–24	0.826	0.333	1.089
25–29	0.616	0.264	0.804
30–34	0.384	0.173	0.497
35–39	0.243	0.172	0.280
40–44	0.058	0.129	0.021
45–49	−0.178	0.033	−0.291
50–54	−0.485	−0.133	−0.673
55–59	−0.774	−0.281	−1.037
60–64	−1.156	−0.522	−1.494
1965	0.368	1.003	0.031
1970	0.701	1.195	0.439
1975	0.626	0.978	0.438
1980	0.490	0.701	0.377
1985	0.287	0.357	0.249
1990	0.218	0.147	0.255
1995	−0.047	−0.258	0.066
2000	−0.737	−1.089	−0.549
2005	−0.794	−1.287	−0.531
2010	−1.112	−1.747	−0.775
1915–19	−0.611	−1.668	−0.048
1920–24	−0.569	−1.486	−0.082
1925–29	−0.500	−1.275	−0.087
1930–34	−0.469	−1.103	−0.131
1935–39	−0.454	−0.948	−0.192
1940–44	−0.448	−0.801	−0.261
1945–49	−0.367	−0.578	−0.254
1950–54	−0.263	−0.333	−0.225
1955–59	−0.135	−0.064	−0.172
1960–64	−0.030	0.181	−0.143
1965–69	0.108	0.460	−0.080
1970–74	0.465	0.958	0.202
1975–79	0.710	1.345	0.373
1980–84	0.763	1.539	0.351
1985–89	0.837	1.753	0.349
1990–94	0.963	2.021	0.401

Note: See text for a description of the basis for these "simulated" results
that are each constrained estimates.

homicide offense rate greater than or at least not less than the 15–19-year-old age category.*

Figure 7.2 displays the results from these three analyses first for the age effects, then for the period effects, and then for the cohort effects. The solid line is the best substantive estimate based on constraining the age curve using substantive knowledge. The dotted line is based on the age1 = age3 constraint that allows the homicide rates for the 15–19-year-olds and 25–29-year-olds to be equal. The dashed line is based on the other boundary solution that allows age4 and age5 to be nearly equal and assures a monotonic decline in the homicide rates after the ages 20–24. The first aim of this approach is

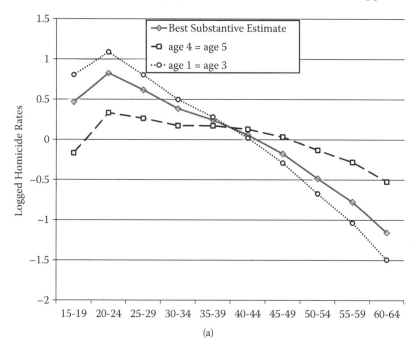

(a)

FIGURE 7.2
Age effects, period effects, and cohort effects based on simulation results using substantive estimates of the age-effects curve for homicide. (a) Age effects. (b) Period effects. (c) Cohort effects. *(continued)*

---

* This does not mean that the homicide rates for those age 15–19 never exceed the rates for those age 25–29. They have done so in the United States since the epidemic of youth homicide. But there are strong reasons to believe that this has been due to the crack cocaine epidemic (Blumstein 1995; Cohen, Cork, Engberg, and Tita 1998; Cork 1999) and to cohort factors such as relative cohort size and the percentage of cohort members born to nonmarried mothers (O'Brien et al. 1999). Note this combination of theory and research (Daly and Wilson 1988; Eisner 2003; Hiraiwa-Hasegawa 2005; Hirschi and Gottfredson 1983; Wilson and Daly 1983) used to justify this constraint.

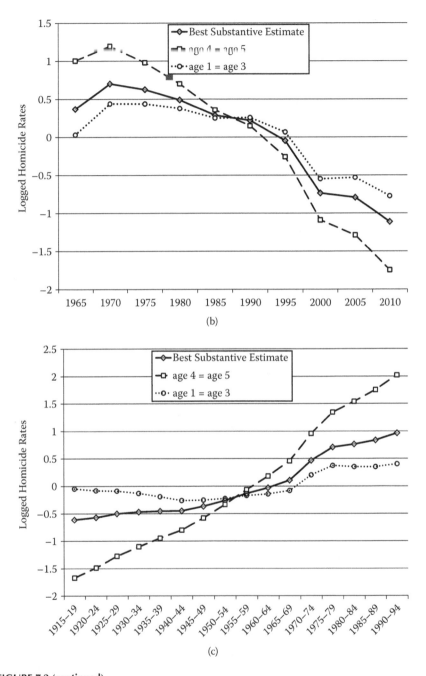

FIGURE 7.2 (continued).
Age effect, period effects, and cohort effects based on simulation results using substantive estimates of the age-effects curve for homicide. (a) Age effects. (b) Period effects. (c) Cohort effects.

that the simulation results for the age curve are credibly in line with substantive knowledge. Examining the age4 = age5 curve indicates that it does not decrease after the age of 20–24 as much as criminologists might expect. Certainly having age group 30–34 and age group 35–39 being almost equal is not expected, even though it meets the monotonic decrease criterion. The age1 = age3 curve shows a steeper monotonic decrease than that portrayed in the age4 = age5 curve. If we do not allow age1 to have a greater age effect than that of age3, then the monotonic decrease should be no greater than that portrayed in the age1 = age3 age curve. Given this, we would expect that the age effects should fall between these two boundaries.

The age curves should seem reasonable, since the best estimate and the boundary estimates are based on substantive knowledge (or expectations). But a major objective in this context of setting these age curves based on substantive knowledge is that if we can produce an accurate age curve in the APC model, then the period and cohort curves should be reasonably accurate. We are using substantive knowledge about something we have some confidence in (the age effects) to tell us something about two factors we have less substantive knowledge about: the period effects and cohort effects. The age-effects curve based on substantive knowledge produces a curve of period effects that would not surprise criminologists. The period curve in Figure 7.2b, based on the best substantive age-curve, shows some fluctuations with a slight downward trend until 1990 when the trend becomes more downward. This corresponds with the great homicide decline that has occurred over the past 20 years as well as the trends for other violent crimes and property crimes as recorded in the Uniform Crime Reports (UCR). What is notable is that this curve is based on fitting the age curve substantively and not on fitting the period curve, which is derivative of the constraint placed on the age-effects curve. The age1 = age3 solution and the age4 = age5 solutions each show this strong period decrease after the 1990 period. The age1 = age3 constraint shows less of a period trend, if any, until after 1990 and the age4 = age5 solution shows a pattern of more negative period effects from the 1970 period forward. This pattern based on the age4 = age5 solution is likely more extreme than expected by criminologists, but it too picks out the great drop in UCR crimes. Each of these simulations indicates an increase in homicide rates from 1965 to 1970 noted by O'Brien (2003), who argues that this surge in violent crime contributed to increased investments in the criminal justice system and eventually led to the war on crime.

More controversial (or simply unknown) in criminology and sociology are the effects of cohorts over time on homicide rates. If the age effects have been constrained reasonably in terms of best substantive knowledge and in terms of the two boundary conditions, then we can gain some knowledge about the trend in cohort effects over time. Using the best estimate there is a linear trend upward in the effects of cohorts over time that is monotonic. The increase is especially apparent after the end of World War II. The age4 = age5 solution shows even more of an increase in the cohort effects over time (the upward slope is greater). The age1 = age3 constrained estimate of the cohort effects does not trend upward (actually slightly downward) until after World War II. Then the cohort effects trend upward until the 1975–79 birth cohort and then are fairly trendless but at a relatively high value in terms of the earlier cohort effects.

Even if we use the two boundary conditions for setting of the age-effects curve for homicide offending, some tentative conclusions can be drawn from this analysis. For example, the overall trend from 1965 to 2010 in the period coefficients is negative. Importantly, the period coefficients have shown a negative and substantial trend since 1990 whether we use the best substantive solution or either of the boundary solutions. The cohort effects for those born in 1915–1919 to 1990–1994 show an overall positive trend. This positive trend is especially marked for the birth cohorts born from 1945–49 to 1990–1994. The change in slope for the birth cohorts 1915–1919 to 1940–1944 and the birth cohorts 1945–1949 to 1990–1994 is an estimable function. It is the same for all constrained solutions, which includes the three solutions in Table 7.3. The slopes for the first set of cohorts and the second set of cohorts are statistically significantly different (p < .001), and the slope for the second set of cohorts is .128 greater than that for the first set of cohorts.

7.2.3 Estimating the Homicide Offending Model with Cohort Characteristics

In this section the homicide offending data is analyzed using two cohort characteristics that were used in Chapter 6 to examine age–period-specific suicide rates in a factor-characteristic model: relative cohort size (RCS) and nonmarital births (NMB). This time, however, the focus is on the relationship of these cohort characteristics to homicide offending and on comparing these results to those based on the s-constraint regression results in the previous section to see if they are consistent with those results. The first column in Table 7.4 contains the results from the age–period (AP) model in which the logged age–period-specific homicide offending rates were regressed on the age and period categorical variables. For the age effects there is a monotonic decrease with age from 20–24 onward. In terms of the hypothesized distribution of age effects, however, the age group 15–19 has an age effect (0.959) that exceeds that for the age group 25–29 (0.830); this does not match the age-effects based on substantive knowledge and theory. But in this situation where the cohort factor has been left out of the model, the age and period categorically coded variables absorb any linear trend in the cohort effects. This model accounts for 95.28% of the variance in the logged age–period-specific homicide offense rates.

TABLE 7.4

Age–Period Model and APCC Model for the Logged Age–Period-Specific Homicide Offending Rate Data

	Age–Period Model Coefficients	APCC Model Coefficients
Intercept	1.856***	–2.191*
15–19	0.986***	0.212
20–24	1.205***	0.643***
25–29	0.866***	0.494***
30–34	0.511***	0.312***
35–39	0.2486***	0.215***
40–44	–0.040	0.071
45–49	–0.348***	–0.096
50–54	–0.741***	–0.350***
55–59	–1.114***	–0.586***
60–64	–1.574 Ref[†]	–0.915 Ref[†]
1965	–0.050	0.610***
1970	0.362***	0.890***
1975	0.371***	0.761***
1980	0.320***	0.571***
1985	0.189*	0.300***
1990	0.224**	0.190***
1995	0.080	–0.119*
2000	–0.487***	–0.859***
2005	–0.415***	–0.977***
2010	–0.592 Ref[†]	–1.367 Ref[†]
ln(RCS)		0.931***
ln(NMB)		1.075***

[*] Significant at.05; ** significant at .01; *** significant at .001 (two-tailed tests).
[†] The coefficients marked Ref are the reference categories for age and period in each of the models.

When the two cohort characteristics are added to the AP model (second column of results), they are each found to be statistically significant at the .001 level. Because both of these independent variables are logged as is the dependent variable, the coefficients can be interpreted as elasticities. A 1% increase in RCS is associated with a 0.931% increase in the age–period-specific homicide offense rates controlling for the other independent variables in the model. A 1% increase in NMB is associated with a 1.075% increase in the age–period-specific homicide rate controlling for the other independent variables in the model. Substantively, these are strong relationships. The percentage of the variance in the logged age–period-specific homicide rates accounted for by this model is 97.97%. This is only a 1.99% increase in the proportion of variance accounted for, but it changes the results for the age and period coefficients significantly by changing their slopes. This occurs, because the trend in the cohort effects over time, as measured by the cohort characteristics, is not zero. In fact, the positive slope in this trend is fairly large as will be shown below.

One last statistic compares the percent of the variance accounted for by cohort characteristics to the percent of variance uniquely accounted for by cohorts. The full APC model accounts for 98.30% of the variance in the age–period-specific homicide rates and the AP model accounts for 95.98% of the variance. That is, the potential amount of additional variance that the cohort characteristics could account for is 2.32%. Adding the cohort characteristics to the AP model accounts for an additional 1.99% of the variance or 85.78% of the variance uniquely accounted for by cohorts [(1.99/2.32) × 100]. Any linear effects that the cohort coefficients might have, however, do not affect this variance accounted for, since the AP model accounts for any linear effects of cohorts. So this measure, though reassuring, does not tell us whether the cohort characteristics have accounted for the linear trend in the cohort effects.

Figure 7.3 compares the results from the APCC analysis with those of the AP model. The AP model constrains the trend in the cohort effect to be zero

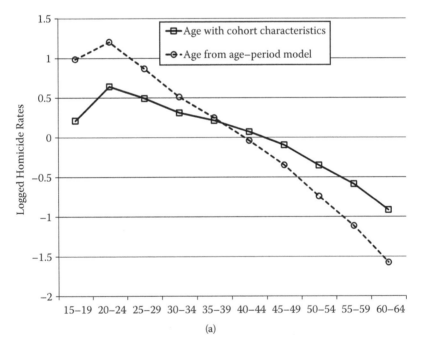

(a)

FIGURE 7.3

Results from the age–period model and the APCC model for the age effects, period effects, and cohort effects. (a) Age effects. (b) Period effects. (c) Cohort effects. *(continued)*

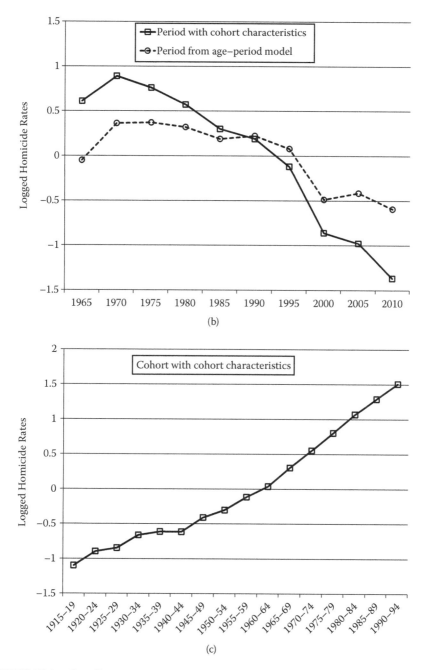

FIGURE 7.3 (continued).
Results from the age–period model and the APCC model for the age effects, period effects, and cohort effects. (a) Age effects. (b) Period effects. (c) Cohort effects.

by not including cohorts in the model. The age and period effects absorb any linear trends in the cohort effects. When cohort characteristics are included they, in a sense, constrain or condition the estimation of the effects of age and period. As can be seen in Figure 7.3c, the cohort effects based on the APCC model display a linear trend that is essentially monotonic and increasing from the birth cohort (1915–1919) to 1990–1994.[*] With the cohort character-istics in the APCC model, they control the age and period effects for this linear trend.

In Figure 7.3a we see that without the cohort characteristics, the AP model (dashed line) indicates that the age effects for those 15–19 are greater than the age effects for those 25–29, which violates the putative relationship based on substantive knowledge. With the cohort characteristics in the model (solid line), however, the age effects fit the substantive criteria. There is a monotonic decrease in the age effects from age 20–24 onward and the rate for 15–19-year-olds is less than that for 25–29-year-olds. Differences in the age effects between the AP model and the APCC model are explained by the cohort effects displayed in Figure 7.3c. Not unexpectedly, since the cohort trend has increased from zero in the AP model to positive in the APCC model (Figure 7.3c) the slope for the age effects has become less negative (more positive) when moving from the AP to APCC model. Correspondingly, the slope for the period effect is more negative in the APCC model than it is in the AP model. The linear components of the solution have been rotated as expected; a solution with a more positive trend in cohorts should result in a more positive slope for ages and a less positive slope for periods.

The final step is to compare the solution based on the substantively gener-ated constraints (best estimate and boundary solutions) and the effects esti-mated by the APCC solution. Those results are summarized in Figure 7.4. Note that the substantively generated *s*-constraint solutions are members of the class of constrained solutions that just identify the APC model. The APCC model with its two cohort characteristics is not one of the least squares solutions to the *full APC model*. But as we have seen, any linear effects of these cohort characteristics shift the trends for the age and period coeffi-cients in a systematic manner. Examining Figure 7.4a shows that the age-effect estimates generated by the cohort characteristics are rather like those of our "best substantive solution" and fit comfortably within the boundaries proposed for plausible substantive solutions. The APCC age-effect estimates (dashed lines with x markings) have a less negative slope than the solution I had selected as the best substantive solution (solid line). The period-effect

---

[*] The cohort effects were calculated in the following manner. Each cohort has its own val-ues of RCS and NMB. We logged these values and multiplied each of them by the logged RCS and logged NMB coefficients in Table 7.4. The sum of these coefficients times their observed values on the cohort characteristics produced the estimated cohort effects. Since the cohort effects based on effect coding are centered on the mean effect, we did the same for these effects. That is, the graph is based on the estimated cohort-effect deviations from the mean of the cohort effects.

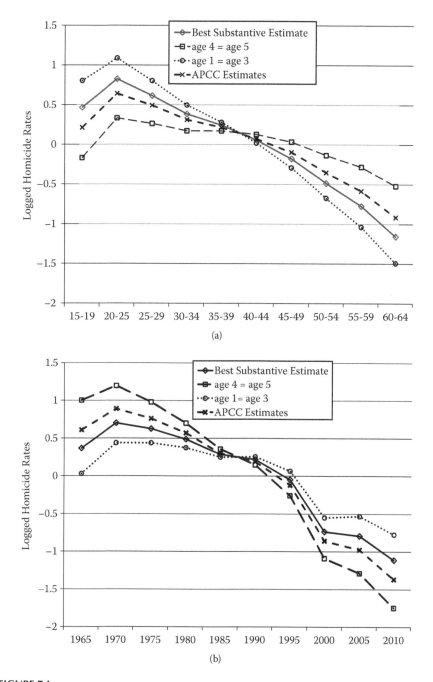

FIGURE 7.4
Best substantive estimates with boundaries to those estimates and APCC estimates. (a) Age effects. (b) Period effects. (c) Cohort effects. *(continued)*

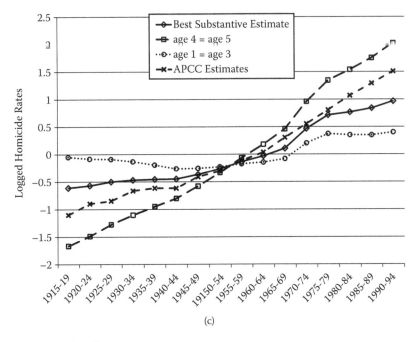

(c)

FIGURE 7.4 (continued).
Best substantive estimates with boundaries to those estimates and APCC estimates. (a) Age effects. (b) Period effects. (c) Cohort effects.

estimates from the APCC model fit comfortably within the plausible substantive solutions generated by the *s*-constraint approach. It has a slightly more negative slope than the "best substantive solution." The cohort-effect estimates based on the APCC model fit within the substantively plausible limits with a somewhat more positive slope than the "best substantive solution." Note that the deviations from the linear trends for the APCC solution do not match exactly with the three (constrained) solutions. For the three constrained solutions those deviations from linearity match exactly, because they are estimable functions.

7.2.4 Conclusions for the Homicide Rate Analysis

In my judgment the strategy outlined in this empirical example is the general sort of tack that those seeking substantive knowledge about the effects of age, period, and cohort from quantitative data should take. That is, there are a variety of analytic tools available, and a number of them have been highlighted in this book. Taken together they can provide some knowledge about the effects of age, period, and cohort. It certainly helps the plausibility of any analysis when different reasonable approaches based on substantive knowledge and theory provide similar results. For example, the difference between the cohort trends for the time period 1915 to 1944 and 1945 to 1994 for the constrained solutions is .128 ($p < .001$). This is an estimable function; it does not depend on the constraint that is used. For the cohort effects based on the two cohort characteristics, the difference in the trends is .125 ($p < .01$) with the trend increasing in both cases for the later cohorts. The cohort characteristics modeled this change in trends almost perfectly; this is reassuring. It builds confidence, but it does not ensure that the overall trend is the same as that for the generating parameters only that the difference in trends within cohorts for these two sets of cohorts is nearly the same.

Using our best substantive estimate for the age effects, the cohort effects trend upwardly monotonically and that is the case for the estimates based on the APCC model (except the upward trend is slightly greater for the APCC-derived cohort effects). The boundary solution in which the age group 15–19 has a rate of homicide offending that is as great as that for those age 25–29 produces an upward trend in the cohort effects overall but not for the first several cohorts.

Equally informative is what these methods tell us about the period effects. The period trend is more downward for the later periods than for the earlier periods. The trends in period effects and the trends in cohort effects are the trends for which there is the least knowledge among criminologists, although most criminologists would not be surprised by the finding that the period effects moved downward from 1990 onward. But for the age effects there is a reasonable amount of agreement. A strength of the proposed method of setting the constraints is that it allows the use the substantive knowledge about something we know more about (the age effects) to gain knowledge about things we know less about, or at least are less certain about: the period and cohort trends.

7.3 Conclusions

The strategies employed in these analyses of homicide arrests involve techniques from several chapters. Tests to see if there are unique nonlinear effects of age, period, and cohort are employed as well as graphs of the deviations from linear trends for the age, period, and cohort effects and shifts of trends within cohorts. These are estimable functions, and they are unbiased estimates of these functions for the parameters that generated the outcome values (Chapters 4 and 5). The point to keep in mind is that we can have the same confidence in these estimable functions as we would have in the individual coefficients from the full APC model itself, if that model were identified.

The s-constraint approach is a "riskier" strategy, since it depends on constrained regression and therefore on how well the constraint is set (Chapters 2 and 3). This technique ameliorates this risk (it does not eliminate it) by setting boundary constraints that seem to be at the edge of plausibility for the effects of the factor for which we have the best substantive knowledge and theory. The final strategy utilized is the factor-characteristic technique (Chapter 6) to estimate the effects of age, period, and cohorts with an age–period–cohort characteristic (APCC) model. This technique produces results that are no better than the characteristics that are used. In the example using homicide offense data, this set of several results employing different approaches is found to provide a consistent and plausible picture of the age, period, and cohort effects for homicide offending over the period 1965 to 2010.

This final empirical example serves more than one purpose. It redisplays some of the techniques examined in this book using an important empirical example. It is also meant to reinforce the importance of using multiple methods when faced with the difficult task of estimation in APC models. The estimable functions provide answers as definitive as any standard identified regression analysis, but they do not answer directly the questions that are typically of greatest interest: that is, what the unbiased estimates are for the individual age, period, and cohort effects that generated the outcome data. The s-constraint regression approach provides direct answers to the question of greatest interest, but the answers need to be based on correct or nearly correct constraints that are no more compelling than the plausibility of the constraints employed. The plausibility of the constraints should be based on strong substantive knowledge and theory. The factor-characteristics approach allows us to assess the role of the characteristics controlling for the two other factors. The coefficients for the two other factors are not particularly compelling unless the characteristics capture the linear trends in the generating parameters for the factor they measure. In this case the linear effects captured by the cohort characteristics produce results that are in line with our best substantive estimates.

This final empirical example is offered in the spirit of Kupper, Janis, Salama, Yoshizawa, and Greenberg (1983: 2803) who note: "Given that the observed Y_{ij}'s are of no help in determining c [the constraint], the only remaining option is to make use of any reasonably reliable a priori, data independent knowledge about the underlying age, period, and cohort effect parameters under study." They then note that constraints should be made on the basis of strong justifications and not based on the data under consideration and that these may be helpful. "If the separate sets of estimates obtained by applying each of these various theoretically-based (a priori) choices are in close agreement, then one could justifiably have some confidence in the accuracy of this common set of estimated age, period, and cohort effects." In this chapter, a set of techniques is used to provide reasonable estimates of the age, period, and cohort effects and the answers they provide are quite consistent. With a view toward methodological modesty and caution, however, I note that these estimates are based on assumptions that include the reasonable shape of the age-effect curve in one case and the adequacy of the cohort characteristics in another.

References

Blumstein, A. 1995. Youth violence, guns and the illicit-drug industry. *Journal of Criminal Law and Criminology* 86:10–36.

Centers for Disease Control and Prevention. 2012. Underlying cause of death 1999-2010 on CDC WONDER. Online Database released 2012, http://wonder.cdc.gov/ucd-icd10.html (accessed Jul 2, 2013), and www.cdc.gov/nchs/data/pop6097

Cohen, J., D. Cork, J. Engberg, and G. Tita. 1998. The role of drug markets and gangs in local homicide rates. *Homicide Studies* 2:241–62.

Cork, D. 1999. Examining space-time interaction in city-level homicide data: Crack markets and the diffusion of guns among youth. 1999. *Journal of Quantitative Criminology* 15:379–406.

Daly, M., and M. Wilson. 1988. *Homicide*. Hawthorne, NY: Aldine de Gruyter.

Easterlin, R. 1978. What will 1984 be like? Socioeconomic implications of recent twists in age structure. *Demography* 15:397–421.

Easterlin, R. 1987. *Birth and Fortune: The Impact of Numbers on Personal Welfare*. Chicago: University of Chicago Press.

Eisner, M. 2003. Long term historical trends in violent crime. *Crime & Justice: A Review of Research* 30: 83–142.

Federal Bureau of Investigation. Various years. *Crime in the United States*. Washington D.C.: Government Printing Office.

Glenn, N.D. 2005. *Cohort Analysis* (2nd edition). Thousand Oaks, CA: Sage.

Hiraiwa-Hasegawa, M. 2005. Homicide by men in Japan, and its relationship to age, resources, and risk taking. *Evolution and Human Behavior* 26:322–43.

Hirschi, T., and M.R. Gottfredson. 1983. Age and the explanation of crime. *American Journal of Sociology* 89:552–84.

Kupper, L.L., J.M. Janis, I.A. Salama, C.N. Yoshizawa, and B.G. Greenberg. 1983. Age-period-cohort analysis: An illustration of the problems in assessing interactions in one observation per cell data. *Communications in Statistics—Theory and Methods* 12:2779–807.

Macunovich, D.J. 1999. The fortunes of one's birth: Relative cohort size and the youth labor market in the United States. *Journal of Population Economics* 12:215–72.

Martin, J.A, B.E. Hamilton, S.J. Ventura, et al. 2012. *Births: Final Data for 2010. National Vital Statistics Reports*, vol. 61 number 1. Hyattsville, MD: National Center for Health Statistics.

O'Brien, R.M. 2003. UCR violent crime rates, 1958–2000: Recorded and offender-generated trends. *Social Science Research*, 32:499–518.

O'Brien, R.M., J. Stockard, and L. Isaacson. 1999. The enduring effects of cohort size and percent of nonmarital births on age-specific homicide rates, 1960–1995. *American Journal of Sociology* 104:1061–95.

Savolainen, J. 2000. Relative cohort size and age-specific arrest rates: A conditional interpretation of the Easterlin effect. *Criminology* 38:117–36.

Stockard, J., and R.M. O'Brien. 2002. Cohort effects on suicide rates: International variations. *American Sociological Review* 67:854–72.

U.S. Bureau of the Census. Various years. Numbers 98, 114, 170, 519, 870, 1000, 1022, 1058, 1127, and for 1995–2010 online. *Current Population Surveys: Series 25.* Washington D.C.: Government Printing Office.

U.S. Bureau of the Census. 1946, 1990. *Vital Statistics of the United States: Natality.* Washington D.C.: Government Printing Office.

Wilson, M., and M. Daly. 1993. A lifespan perspective on homicidal violence: The young male syndrome. In *Proceedings of the 2nd Annual Workshop of the Homicide Research Working Group*, ed. C.R. Block and R.L. Block, 29–38. Washington D.C.: National Institute of Justice.

Yang, Y., W.J. Fu, and K.C. Land. 2004. A methodological comparison of age-period-cohort models: Intrinsic estimator and conventional generalized linear models. In *Sociological Methodology*, ed. R.M. Stolzenberg, 75–110. Oxford: Basil Blackwell.

Yang, Y., S. Schulhofer-Wohl, W.J. Fu, and K.C. Land. 2008. The intrinsic estimator for age-period-cohort analysis: What it is and how to use it. *American Journal of Sociology* 113:1697–736.

Index